total
core
fitness

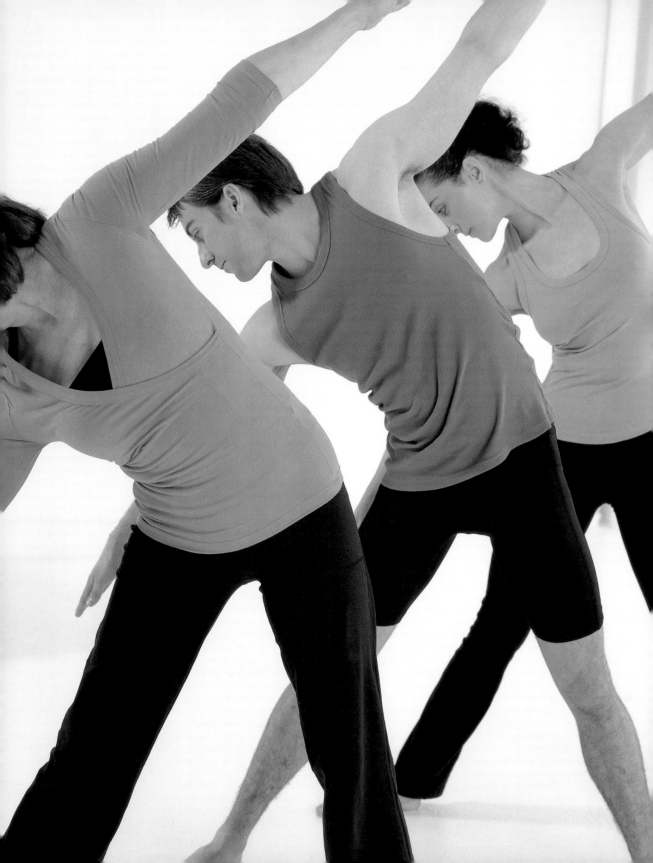

total core fitness

Stronger, leaner, and fitter to the core

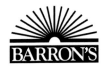

BARRON'S

First edition for the United States, and its dependencies
published in 2006 by Barron's Educational Series, Inc.

Copyright © Elwin Street Limited 2006

All inquiries should be addressed to:
Barron's Educational Series, Inc.
250 Wireless Boulevard
Hauppauge, New York 11788
www.barronseduc.com

Library of Congress Catalog Card No.: 2005924645
ISBN-13: 9780-7641-3321-3
ISBN-10: 0-7641-3321-7

Conceived and produced by
Elwin Street Limited
79 St John Street
London EC1M 4NR
www.elwinstreet.com

Designer: Louise Leffler
Photographer: Mike Prior
Models: Amy Corey, Kathy Corey, Paul Williams
Clothes and equipment supplied by Sweaty Betty, Bloch,
Fitness Network, and Kathy Corey

Printed and bound in Singapore
9 8 7 6 5 4 3 2 1

While every effort has been made to ensure
that the content of this book is technically
accurate and as sound as possible,
neither the author nor the publishers
can accept responsibility for any
injury or loss sustained as a result
of this material.

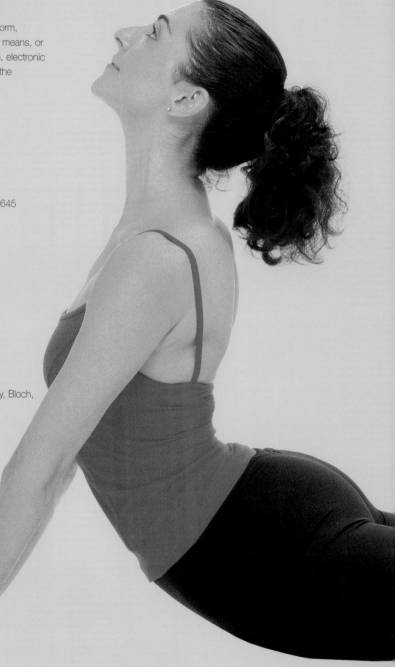

Contents

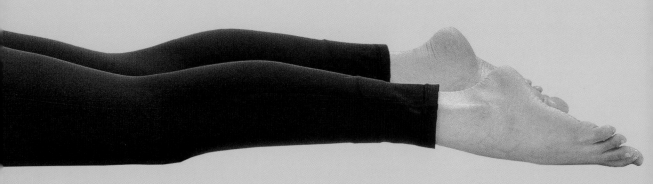

THE GOAL IS TO ENRICH YOUR QUALITY OF LIFE.
IMPROVED HEALTH, WELL-BEING, STRENGTH, AND
FLEXIBILITY ARE ALL WITHIN YOUR REACH.

Introduction

Wouldn't you like to go to bed at night and wake up feeling fitter in the morning? That is the purpose of this book. Designed to create a more efficient way for your body to function, this is unlike any other fitness program. The emphasis is not on exercise, repetitions, or building muscles, and the goals are not to increase the numbers of sets, reps, or weights. The goal of this program is to enrich your quality of life with a fitter and more functional body that moves fluidly and performs daily activities with more ease. Improved health, well-being, strength, and flexibility are all within your reach.

The results of a fitness program depend on the specific type of work and how hard and often you work out. This means that both the quantity and quality of the exercises affect the outcome. In the past the "more is better" and "no pain, no gain" approach dominated the exercise world. These attitudes are in direct conflict with the latest research in the fields of exercise physiology and sports medicine. The recommendations of three intense workouts per week with days of rest in between have been replaced with recommendations of mild-to-moderate exercise on most if not every day of the week. If we look

Kathy Corey,
Master Teacher of the Pilates Method

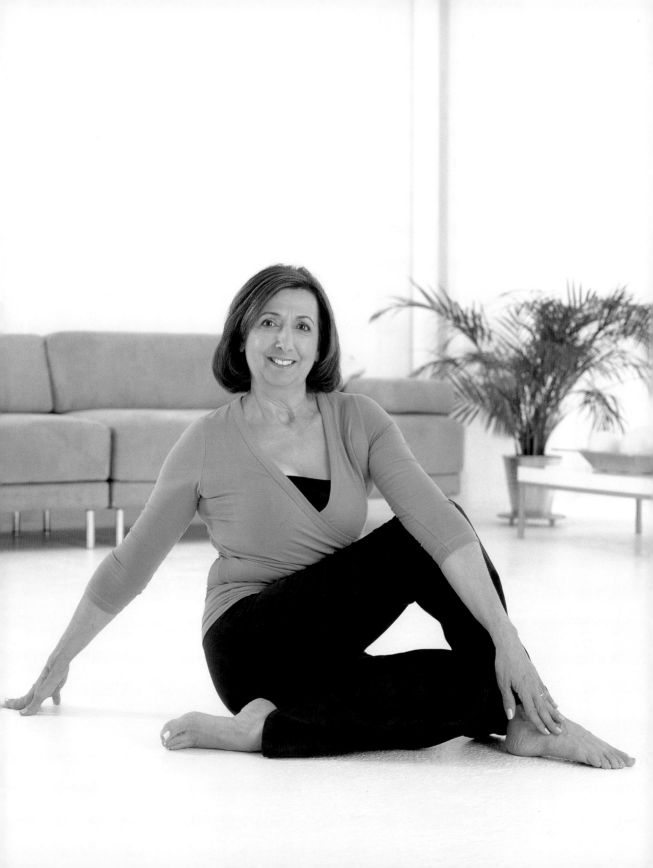

logically at this shift in approach, it makes perfect sense. You don't go to work three days a week and stay in bed on the other days, or eat only every other day. Life is a continuous interplay of mental and physical activity, rest, and action.

With new goals in mind, these exercise programs have been designed to improve daily physical fitness, because when we are in better shape, we change the shape of our lives. An increase in physical fitness improves physical activity. Practical fitness makes life easier and more fun.

However, it works only to the extent that you make it work, for what you do with your body in the time that you are not exercising is more important to your overall flexibility, strength, and fitness than the hours spent working out. The way you stand, walk, sleep, and breathe will have a greater effect on your physical well-being than any exercise program.

But this book is about much more than exercise. It shows you how to make a conscious choice to live a healthy lifestyle that embraces a holistic approach to life and takes responsibility for personal health. Through this program, you will first acquire control of your core muscles and then progress to a natural rhythm that connects to all mental and subconscious activities. This process replaces misaligned physical habits with realigned patterns. It is a twenty-four-hour-a-day fitness program. It is movement for life.

My approach combines a variety of time-tested techniques into a single program. These methods complement one another in the same way that the varied activities of our days interact with one another. Repetitive activity and overuse leads to boredom and both mental and physical strain. Living in the "information age" offers us the ability to understand and experience the mind-body connection more fully than ever before. The approach in this book draws on both Eastern and Western exercise regimens and synthesizes them with the most current physiological research to create a program that energizes and balances your body as you improve your posture, alignment, breathing, circulation, strength, and flexibility.

In order to simulate the specific movements you use in daily activities, many different exercise techniques are necessary. The best moves from Pilates, stability ball work, yoga, and weight training have been compiled here and programmed in specific order to balance complementary muscle groups for maximum efficiency. This plan is like having a personal trainer in your home because it allows anybody at any level of fitness to work at their maximum potential. If you are a novice, you will engage your core muscles right from the start for greater results. If you are an athlete, you will add more precision to your workout, doing less work for a superior outcome.

Concentration and careful movement make this program a mind-body approach to exercise. This program creates a core of strength from which all movements, from simple walking to intense athletics, are generated. Using your core makes your body, mind, and life more centered and balanced. Alignment, control, and focus are your secrets to success. These principles are essential to your workout, because without complete attention to the movement process, you won't be able to achieve results as deeply or as quickly.

A hundred years ago, the average life expectancy was forty-seven years. Today, in most Western countries, it is close to eighty. But what we have not yet obtained is the quality of life that needs to be consistent with the quantity of life. Enjoying life requires a healthy body. In the journey from birth to youth then aging, the balance of mental and physical energy combined with the joy of life is the gift of being.

The ideal body is one that moves with fluidity, grace, and a fusion of strength and balance. With concentration and dedication to the performance of core fitness, the ideal body is yours.

WHAT YOU DO WITH YOUR BODY IN THE TIME THAT YOU ARE NOT EXERCISING IS MORE IMPORTANT TO YOUR OVERALL FLEXIBILITY, STRENGTH, AND FITNESS THAN THE HOURS SPENT WORKING OUT.

How Core Fitness Works

Your core holds you up and is called upon whenever you move, stretch, twist, or walk. It is your strength center and the source of aches and pains if you don't treat it right.

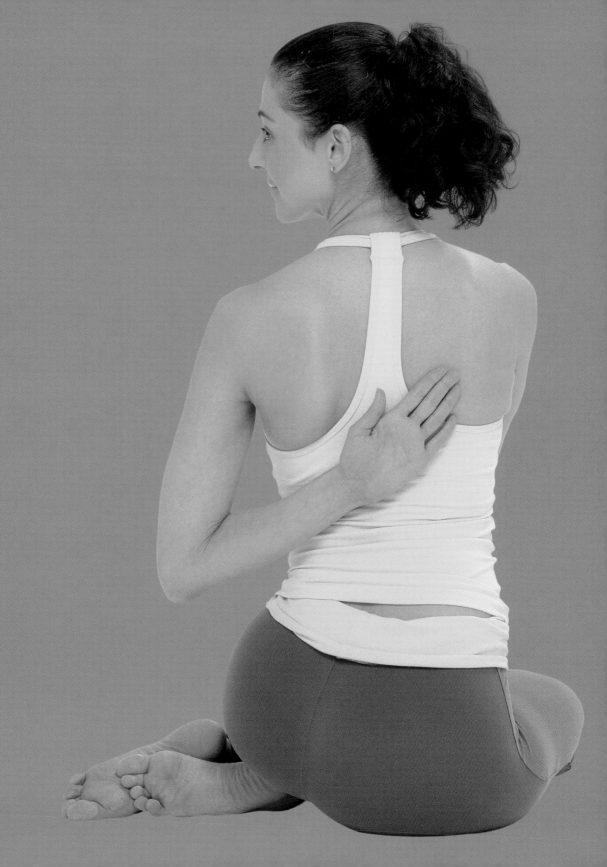

Why train your core muscles?

Your core is your power or strength center. It includes the muscles in your torso at your back, sides, and abdomen. No matter where your aches and pains occur, the source of the problem can generally be found in the body's core, and correcting these problems at their source is the only way to eliminate them. The core bones, muscles, and organs from your tailbone and pelvis to your shoulders and neck determine whether your movements are in balance or if you are an injury in the making.

Think of your body as a machine. All the parts need to work harmoniously for the machine to run smoothly. And the performance of any machine requires maintenance and care. Without good care you can begin a cycle that leads to strain and injury. Since ideal alignment is crucial for optimal movement, the more precise your alignment, the better the performance of the rest of your body.

The way you lift and carry everything, from your books to your baby or your briefcases, creates your personal movement habits. Like fingerprints, each individual has their own characteristic pattern. You may lift with your biceps at the front of your arms; I may lift with my upper trapezius muscles on top of my shoulders. These movement patterns, when repeated over time, alter how you work—and how you look. Swinging a golf club, tennis racquet, or baseball bat, if not done in the correct alignment, will cause muscle imbalances and joint impairments.

The techniques and exercises in this book work the body from the inside out. They address only the quantity of movement, but also the quality of life.

WHAT ARE YOUR PERSONAL MOVEMENT HABITS? THESE MOVEMENTS, WHEN REPEATED OVER TIME, ALTER HOW YOU WORK—AND HOW YOU LOOK.

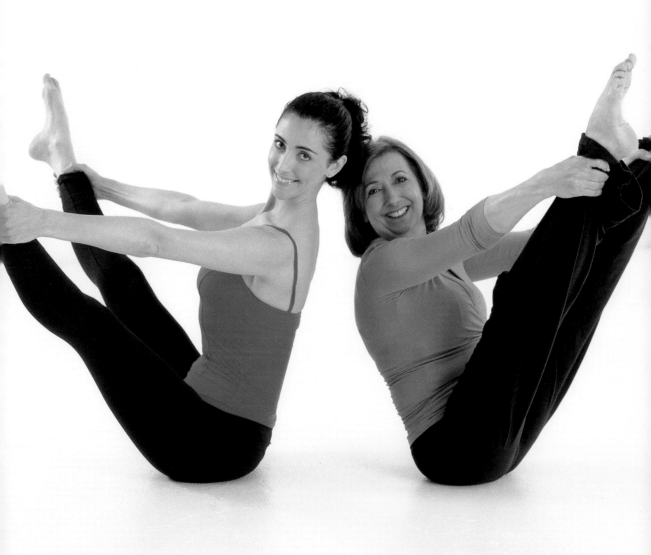

What makes up your core?

Anatomy is like learning a new language for your body. This reference guide explains the key muscle groups to help make the exercises work for your full benefit.

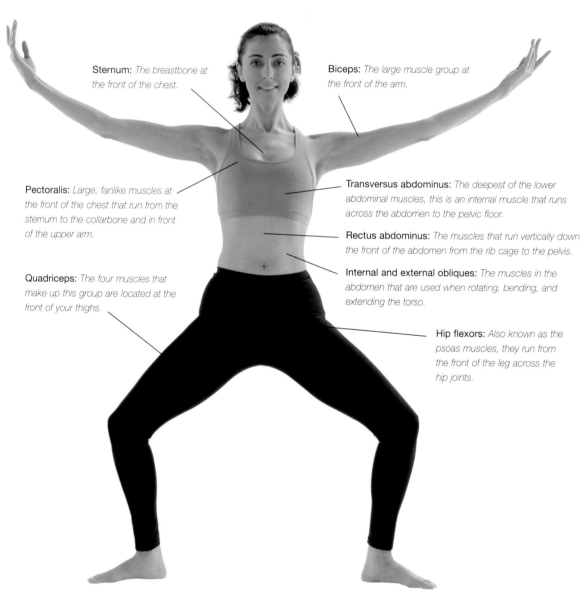

Sternum: *The breastbone at the front of the chest.*

Biceps: *The large muscle group at the front of the arm.*

Pectoralis: *Large, fanlike muscles at the front of the chest that run from the sternum to the collarbone and in front of the upper arm.*

Transversus abdominus: *The deepest of the lower abdominal muscles, this is an internal muscle that runs across the abdomen to the pelvic floor.*

Rectus abdominus: *The muscles that run vertically down the front of the abdomen from the rib cage to the pelvis.*

Internal and external obliques: *The muscles in the abdomen that are used when rotating, bending, and extending the torso.*

Quadriceps: *The four muscles that make up this group are located at the front of your thighs.*

Hip flexors: *Also known as the psoas muscles, they run from the front of the leg across the hip joints.*

Cervical: *The first seven vertebrae in the neck. This is the most flexible section of your spine.*

Rhomboids: *Thin muscles in the back, along the spine, that are responsible for moving the shoulder blades.*

Shoulder girdle: *The muscles surrounding the shoulder joints.*

Trapezius: *A long, triangular muscle that runs from the neck and shoulders to the base of the thoracic spine.*

Scapula: *The shoulder blades.*

Triceps: *Three muscles that make up the only muscle in the back of the upper arm.*

Thoracic vertebrae: *The twelve vertebrae from the bottom of the neck through the rib cage, in the upper to middle sections of your back. The twelve ribs are attached to these vertebrae.*

Deltoids: *The triangular muscle of the shoulder that passes up and over the shoulder joint.*

Latissimus dorsi: *Large, fanlike muscles in the back that attach to the arms, vertebrae, and pelvis.*

Lumbar vertebrae: *The five vertebrae in the lower back. They are larger and have limited mobility.*

Gluteus: *Maximus, minimus, and medius are the buttock muscles, the largest muscle group and considered the strongest in the body.*

Sacrum vertebrae: *The five fused vertebrae in the lower back.*

Hamstrings: *The large muscle group at the back of the upper thigh.*

Coccyx: *The tailbone; the lowest four vertebrae, which are also fused into one bone.*

Your core

The frame

Your pelvis, hip bones, rib cage, and shoulder girdle create the frame and central support of your core. Your core muscles, tendons, and ligaments form the links that hold this frame together, providing both stability and mobility for the whole body. This vital system must work harmoniously with a balance of strength and flexibility for the rest of your body to function properly.

The powerhouse

Your abdominal muscles attach your upper body to your lower body. They transmit the power necessary for all movement, from the turn of your head to the curl of your toes. Consisting of four layers of muscles that crisscross your torso, they support your spine, organs, and pelvis. They keep you upright and are responsible for your breathing. Whole-body function is dependent on the balance and counterbalance of this complex internal system.

The transversus abdominus, the deepest layer of abdominals, encircles your waist horizontally and is attached to your diaphragm. It plays an important role in your breathing, supporting your organs and stabilizing your spine and pelvis.

If properly working, the transversus abdominus contracts before your arms and legs move to stabilize your spine and pelvis. If your spine is unstable, your nervous system will not recruit the extremity muscles efficiently and your movements will be unbalanced.

For your movements to be in balance, these four muscle groups must also be in balance. Working the superficial layer, the topmost layer that is used in most exercise programs, can actually create less balance between muscle groups, diminishing their work as a unit. Working from your core, from the inside out, creates a system of functional strength and improves the efficiency of all movement.

Lifting and bending

The rectus abdominus, also known as the "six-pack" muscle, runs vertically from your rib cage to your pubic bone. It aids in lifting and bending forward, and is a prime mover in helping to get you from lying down to standing up.

The internal and external obliques run diagonally down the sides of your body. Not only do they work with the rectus abdominus in forward bending, but they are also responsible for rotational movements.

The support structures

The pelvic floor spans the area underneath the pelvis and plays a primary role in supporting the contents of the pelvis and abdominal wall. Pelvic alignment affects all movements through your legs and feet, and all movements from your legs and feet affect the alignment of the pelvis. This symbiotic relationship means problems of misalignment will occur anywhere that the kinetic chain has a weak link. Keeping your core connections strong builds strong links.

Your rib cage attaches to the thoracic spine and encircles the torso to attach to the breastbone in the front. This structure has the ability to expand and contract by three full inches on inhalation and exhalation; however, if you do not take advantage of this mobility, it becomes rigid and loses flexibility. Your ribs are multidirectional, with the capability of moving up, down, forward, and back. Your rib cage has the ever-important job of protecting your heart and lungs and is vital to your breathing.

The spine

The ideal spine needs to be both stable and very mobile to fulfill its varied functions. It works as an intermediary between the upper and lower body and supports the weight of your head, organs, and limbs. It also protects your spinal cord.

The vertebral column consists of twenty-four separate vertebrae, the sacrum, and the coccyx. The cervical spine consists of seven vertebrae

WORKING FROM YOUR CORE, FROM THE INSIDE OUT, IMPROVES THE EFFICIENCY OF ALL MOVEMENT.

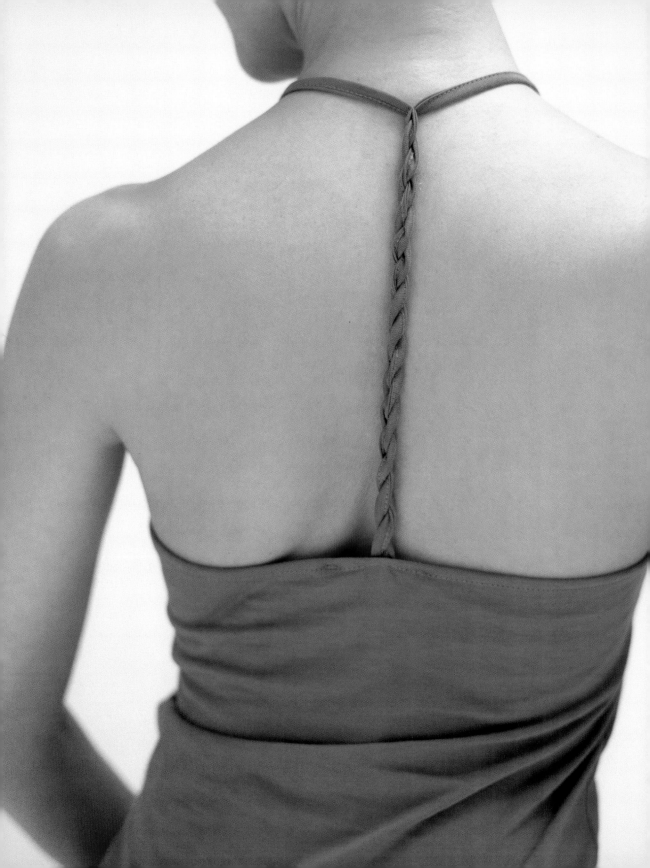

and is the highest and most mobile part of the spine. The thoracic spine consists of twelve vertebrae that attach to the rib cage. Five large vertebrae compose the lumbar spine in the lower section of the back. The base of the spine is called the sacrum. It is composed of five fused vertebrae. The coccyx or tailbone consists of the lowest four vertebrae, which are also fused into one bone.

You are born with your primary curve, the thoracic curve. Your opposing curves, necessary to sit, stand, and walk, are developed by your first movements. The curve in the cervical spine develops as an infant lifts its head to explore the surrounding world. Kicking, rolling, and crawling produce the curvature in the lumbar spine.

The position of the bones in your pelvis influences the curvature of your spine. Excessive forward tilt of the top of your pelvis increases your lumbar curve in your lower back, which in turn increases the other curves. A greater degree of curvature makes your individual vertebrae less well aligned on top of one another, increasing the stresses at the joints of your spinal column. If you work on proper placement of the pelvis, you'll reduce these curves and stresses.

However, a back that is too straight is also not ideal, because it absorbs less shock. If you tuck your pelvis in to straighten the curve of your back, you distort the alignment of your legs and increase tension in your pelvis. This impedes the functioning of your pelvic muscles and reduces the efficiency of your hip joints. A balanced pelvis is based on good movement patterns, and becomes a part of the way we move, sit, and stand.

THE IDEAL SPINE NEEDS TO BE BOTH STABLE AND VERY MOBILE TO FULFILL ITS VARIED FUNCTIONS. IT WORKS AS AN INTERMEDIARY BETWEEN YOUR UPPER AND LOWER BODY.

The way to core fitness

"Overload" and "specificity"

The major principles of exercise touted by fitness experts are "overload" and "specificity." Overload works your muscles, exposing them to a load greater than they are normally accustomed to. Repeating this exposure improves functional capacity. The interaction of the intensity of your workout with how long and how often you exercise results in cumulative overload. Progress is made as your body adapts to a greater load and you achieve new fitness goals.

The principle of specificity says that results are specific to the muscles being trained. Overload to your biceps will build only your biceps. To increase functional strength and achieve core fitness, you will work your whole body in a balanced, holistic way. The more muscle groups involved in performing a single movement, the more efficient your movements will be. Engagement of your core makes all movements, even your biceps curls and calf raises, core exercises.

Creating a system in which your muscles work together and support one another lessens muscle fatigue and decreases the chance of injury. Activating this system before contracting specific muscles makes movement more efficient.

Different types of muscle contractions

Fitness experts and physical therapists use a few useful terms when talking about different types of exercises and contractions:

Isotonic concentric contraction: Contractions that permit the muscles to shorten

Isotonic eccentric contraction: The active lengthening of muscles in activity

Isometric contraction: Muscles are activated and held at a constant length

Passive stretch: Muscles are lengthened in a passive state and are not being stimulated to contract

THE MORE MUSCLE GROUPS INVOLVED IN PERFORMING A SINGLE MOVEMENT, THE MORE EFFICIENT YOUR MOVEMENTS WILL BE.

You use all of these types of contractions every day without knowing it. If you lift a box and carry it across the room, place it on a table, and then put it on the floor, you have just completed all of the above contractions. Lifting the box is a concentric contraction because it shortens the muscles toward the body. Carrying the box across the room is an isometric contraction because you are holding the box at a constant length. Placing the box on a table works your muscles eccentrically as they lengthen to allow you to put it down. Lowering the box to the floor stretches your hamstrings in a passive stretch as they release in order for you to bend down.

Open chain and closed chain exercises

Exercises are also classified as "open chain" or "closed chain." In an open chain exercise the end that is the farthest away from your body is not in contact with a stable surface. When you lift your leg off the floor it becomes an open chain. Biceps curls, standing single leg circles, and back extension exercises are all in this category. This form of exercise strengthens one set of muscles and is very specific in training that muscle group.

Closed chain exercises have your extremity in contact with a stable surface at the farthest end. Push-ups, lunges, and standing knee bends are in this group. This type of exercise strengthens several muscle groups simultaneously and creates movements that are more functional.

Combinations to achieve total core fitness

The combination of isotonic and isometric contractions with closed chain and open chain exercises creates a balanced program that uniformly develops your body. Since these movements are done in a controlled manner on a daily basis with this program, every movement during your day becomes a core movement.

Keeping your core aligned

Core alignment begins at your hips and pelvis. Their position determines the curvature of the lower back and the amount of muscle work necessary to perform each movement. Too much or too little curve creates a greater risk of injuring your back.

The top of your core is at your shoulders and chest. The forward hunch of your shoulders or the thrust of your rib cage also throws your body out of alignment. Therefore the relationship between your hips and shoulders is crucial to how your muscles work.

Starting at your hips, imagine a line coming through your body from side to side. Imagine a second line coming through front to back. The cross point of those two lines in the center of your pelvis creates your pelvic alignment. The ideal standing position is to keep the cross point level and equal in the center of your pelvis. To do this, pull your muscles toward your joints, pulling them evenly inward. This will prevent the sway or arch of the back and the tuck of your pelvis.

Contract your lower abdominal muscles and pull your navel to your spine. Lengthen the space in your torso between your hip bones and rib cage to activate your deeper layers of muscles.

Imagine two more lines coming in front-to-back and side-to-side at your shoulders and chest. Hold this second cross point equal and level to prevent slouching your shoulders or arching your upper back.

Your third cross point comes in at your ears, nose, and back of your head. The even placement of this cross point prevents your head from jutting forward or arching your neck.

For correct alignment, draw an imaginary vertical line through all three cross points and have them remain aligned over one another. This posture activates all the core muscles in a balanced way that prevents fatiguing one muscle group at the expense of another.

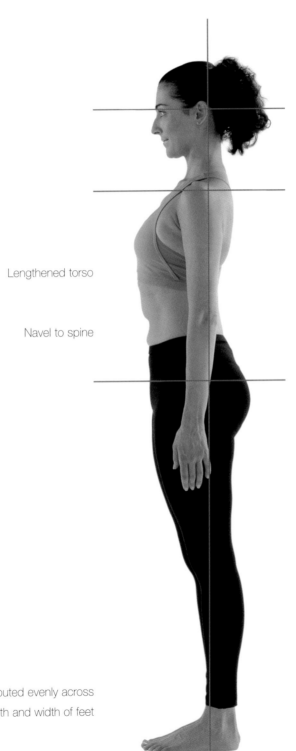

Lengthened torso

Navel to spine

Weight distributed evenly across
length and width of feet

Foot placement

Your core alignment is also dependent upon your foot placement. Think about each foot as a triangle. The triangle runs from under your big toe across to your little toe and back to the center of your heel. Distribute your body weight evenly into these triangles to prevent rolling in or out on your feet. Your legs should be straight. Make sure not to lock or rotate your knees but to keep them pointing straight forward to maintain your alignment.

Connect the energy from your foot triangles through your legs to your hips, shoulders, and head.

Neutral spine and imprinted spine

Core alignment includes working with what's called a "neutral spine" and an "imprinted spine." Your neutral spine is your most lengthened spine, allowing for maximum motion in all directions, and the spaces for the spinal nerves are in a more opened position. Imprinting your spine is the process of pressing the full length of your spine down, one vertebra at a time. This creates an "imprint" of each vertebra by stretching and elongating the spine. In both of these positions, your pelvis is not tucked, which tightens the hip flexors and buttock muscles.

IF YOU INCORPORATE CORE ALIGNMENT INTO EVERY EXERCISE, YOU WILL REDUCE THE CHANCES OF INJURY AND INCREASE THE EFFECTIVENESS OF THE MOVEMENT.

For a neutral spine, do not arch your back or flatten your back to the floor. The natural curve of your spine should still be present.

The concept of neutral spine plays an essential role in core alignment. Think of your pelvis as a bowl filled to the very top with water. If the bowl tips to the front, the water will spill out the front of the bowl. If it tilts too far back, the water will run out the back. This concept holds true for any place on the circumference of the bowl. If the bowl is held stable, the contents will remain intact. If you place the structure of the pelvis in its neutral position, the surrounding muscles, joints, and tendons will have less work to do to keep the bowl steady and not spill any of the imaginary water. This key core positioning sets the placement for the rest of your alignment and is the foundation of core fitness.

Shoulder and rib cage placement

The structure and function of the shoulder girdle and rib cage completes the upper section of your core alignment. Proper shoulder alignment is crucial for the movement of your arms, neck, and head.

The correct placement for your sternum should be neither tipped upward nor downward, but vertical at the front of your chest. Shoulder placement needs to be centered; arching or slouching impedes the efficient functioning of your shoulders.

How core fitness affects movements in your arms and legs

Core alignment integrates the body as a whole. The interrelationship of your body segments to your core creates balance in movement. Using core structure to align and activate the whole body to perform movement creates your system of functional strength.

Movement is most efficient when it passes through the center of your joints. Alignment of your shoulders will make your golf swing more powerful; alignment of your hips and pelvis will improve how you walk. Incorporating core alignment into every exercise, especially exercises for the arms and legs, reduces the chance of injury and increases the effectiveness of the movement.

Balancing the best techniques

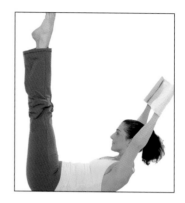

Pilates

Joseph Hubertus Pilates was a visionary—a man ahead of his time. Born near Düsseldorf, Germany, in 1880, he was a sickly child. To improve his health, he studied both Eastern and Western exercise techniques including yoga, Zen, and ancient Roman and Greek regimens.

The exercise technique he developed, named after him, is a mind-body system that uses the whole body to develop strong, flexible, and well-toned muscles. The Pilates Method is founded on the principal connection between concentration and activity. The technique brings focus to each movement pattern so that the mind directly shapes the body.

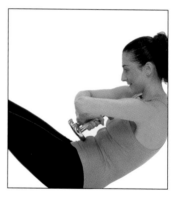

Pilates is based on the principle that a few movements, performed accurately and with control, are worth more than hundreds of mindless repetitions. To be performed properly, each and every exercise in the program must include all of the following elements: concentration, control, centering, precision, flow of movement, and breathing.

Weight training

Weight training tends to target individual muscle groups rather than integrate the whole body to perform the movement. Most weight-training exercises emphasize working one or two muscle groups and separating the programs into upper-body or lower-body workouts. This type of program usually allows for a day of rest after working the specific muscle group. Weight training loads specific muscle groups, exposing them to more weight than they are used to. Repeating the weight training movements improves the strength of the specific muscle group.

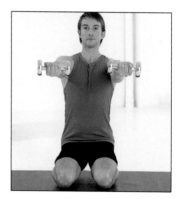

In this book you'll find the best weight training moves often combined with moves from other regimens.

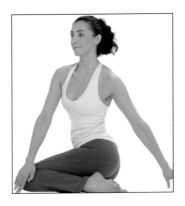

Yoga

Dating back more than five thousand years, yoga has its roots in ancient India, and it is both a physical and spiritual practice. There are many different types of yoga, including Ashtanga, Iyengar, and Bikram, but all use a series of set movements called "poses" as a way of stretching, toning, and strengthening the body. Like Pilates, the focus is on controlled movement and awareness of what is going on in the body. Yoga is a mental and physical process that rejuvenates and energizes the system on all levels.

In the workout programs that follow, the Sanskrit names appear along with the common English names for yoga poses.

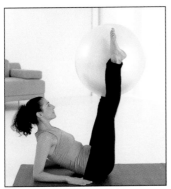

Stability ball

A more recent development to the fitness world, the stability ball was originally created as an aid for physical therapy. Because it is is an unstable base, it requires more muscle groups to work simultaneously. Every exercise becomes a balancing act, which makes concentration a necessary part of each movement. Stability-ball work improves coordination, and activates and stabilizes your muscles.

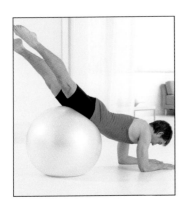

Combining "the best of the best"

Although each technique works differently, the goals are the same: achieving a higher level of fitness. Blending the techniques produces the results you use every day. You do not stay in bed today because yesterday was your "leg exercise day" and today you can work only your arms. You do not reach for a pen at your office and stay there for five inhalations and five exhalations. Each technique must find its most useful path to allow greater freedom of movement in your life. The program shifts from Pilates to stability ball, weight training, and yoga for faster results. The sequence of the movement patterns creates a biomechanical rhythm of energy, strength, and power. The programs in this book create an environment for you to experience more fully what you take for granted every day—the joy of movement, the joy of life.

The role of the breath

Breath is your body's fuel and its nourishment. This all-important delivery of oxygen affects your simplest daily tasks, your intense physical activities, and your emotional stress. Breath is your vital mind-body connection.

Your lungs can hold up to five quarts of air, but as you age, this capacity decreases. Less surface area is used, and your lungs begin to shut down. The small muscles that connect your ribs become weak and lose the ability to work efficiently. You then end up using only the upper portion of your lungs.

Traditionally, two types of breathing techniques have been employed in fitness regimens, and we're going to combine the best of each.

Thoracic breathing

Your rib cage has the ability to expand and contract three full inches with each breath. Thoracic breathing opens and closes your rib cage at both the front and the back of your chest, stimulating the small muscles to expand and contract with ease and fluidity.

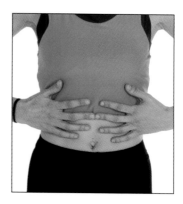

To feel thoracic breathing, place your hands on your rib cage with your fingers touching at the center of your chest. Inhale through your nose, allowing your rib cage to expand and your hands to separate. Exhale through your mouth and feel your rib cage close inward as your hands come together once again.

Diaphragmatic breathing

The walls of the abdomen are composed of three muscular sheets. Forming the top of the abdominal-pelvic cavity is the thoracic diaphragm. The thoracic diaphragm is attached to the rib cage in the front and to the lumbar vertebrae in the back, and domes upward into the thoracic cavity.

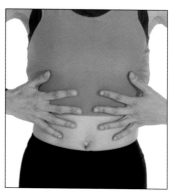

On an inhalation, your thoracic diaphragm contracts and lowers, increasing the volume of the thoracic cavity. At the same time, the diaphragm presses down on the abdominal cavity, massaging your internal organs and aiding in the return of blood to your heart.

To perform diaphragmatic breathing, place your hands on your abdomen just below your navel. Inhale deeply and slowly exhale. Inhale again and exhale through your mouth, contracting your lower abdominal muscles. Feel your abdomen pull inward as the contraction pushes more air out of your lungs. This method of breathing makes every exhalation an abdominal exercise and will help to tone and flatten your abdominal muscles.

Core breathing

Combining thoracic and diaphragmatic breathing principles improves lung capacity and increases the oxygenation of the red blood cells. In traditional workouts, the deep abdominal muscles are not consciously exercised until you attain a very high level of fitness. But with core breathing, each breath becomes an internal strengthening exercise that improves lung function, flattens your abdomen, and integrates more of the body.

Core breathing matches the movement of the exercises to the way you inhale and exhale. To perform this breathing exercise, place your hands on your rib cage with your fingers touching at the center of your chest. Inhale through your nose, allowing your chest to expand, and watch your fingers stretch apart, noting the amount of space between them. Exhale through your mouth, and allow your fingers to touch at the center of your chest. As your fingers come together, pull your lower abdominal muscles inward to fully expel the air from your lungs.

Now, divide the inhalation into two parts, bringing in a greater amount of air. Exhale through your mouth in two parts. Repeat the exercise dividing the inhalations and exhalations into three parts, then four parts, and then five parts. Watch the space between your fingers grow as you increase the number of inhalations, expanding your chest and developing your lung capacity.

If you practice this breathing daily, you will be able to develop your chest expansion and improve your circulation. Performing core breathing while you exercise also helps to prevent the build-up of toxins in your system and energizes body and mind.

"BREATHING IS OUR FIRST ACT OF LIFE, AND OUR LAST." JOSEPH PILATES

Progressing through the programs using maximum potential

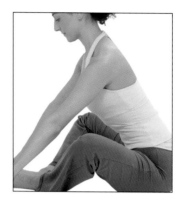

The first program, "Putting the Principles to Work," is for everyone, no matter what your level of fitness. It will help set your alignment, focus, and concentration for the programs that follow, "Dynamic Strength Training" and "The Total Core Challenge." In order to progress from program to program, use the following guidelines:

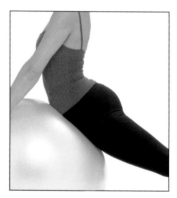

✻ For your work with weights, complete three sets of repetitions with a heavy weight before progressing to the next level.

✻ For yoga poses, maintain the pose without the aid of a strap or lock for the full length of time recommended.

✻ For your Pilates exercises, you should be able to perform the movements with precision and flow of motion.

✻ For your stability ball exercises, you should be able to maintain your balance and not use momentum to complete the movements.

When you feel confident that you have achieved the maximum work from program 1, progress to program 2, and so on. And if you get bored with the pattern of the three programs that form the bulk of the book, turn to pages 150–155, where you will find a variety of mix-and-match workouts to suit your everyday needs. From a 10-minute stretching workout to a full and challenging 60-minute session, you can enjoy a daily program that fits your fitness level and your lifestyle.

But whatever program you begin, remember that the aim is to work to your individual maximum potential. The concept of working to

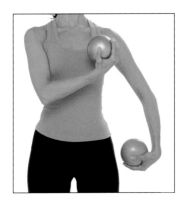

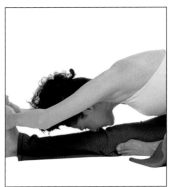

maximum potential is not about how many sit-ups you can do in a minute, how much weight you can bench-press, or even how fast you can complete a marathon. Exercise, like most things in life, has a dose-response relationship. Too much or too little lacks balance. Some exercise is better than no exercise, but only up to a point is more better than less. Like a good meal leaves you feeling satisfied, an exercise program should leave you feeling invigorated, not depleted. If you are working your body to the point of fatigue, you are passing the point where more is better. Supersized exercise is just not necessary. Why overwork your muscles when you don't need to?

Maximum potential should challenge your mind as well as your body, since to be truly fit, the mind-body connection needs to be exercised. Exercise should improve physical fitness and lead to an improvement in all physical activity and the ability to enjoy a long, healthy life.

The concept of maximum potential is also an individual thing. You are working to your maximum potential if you are performing the movements in the correct alignment, with concentration, and precision. Challenge yourself to work more deeply and more slowly. Keep in mind the following pointers and you'll be well on the way to developing dynamic core strength:

* If you are truly using core strength, you should be able to stop at any point in an exercise and hold that position or even reverse the movement.

* If you cannot follow the breathing pattern as described in each exercise, you are using too much weight or your body's momentum to complete the exercise. Be sure to keep the breathing pattern throughout the exercise.

* Keep your form as you perform the movements, and remember that your alignment and positioning are more important than how many repetitions you perform or how much weight you use.

Questions and answers about the equipment

Why use a resistance band?

The use of a resistance band means you are working opposing forces in the exercises, which stabilizes core joints so that you can increase their mobility. This stretch-and-strengthen technique offers optimum muscle work while lubricating your joints. Use a Core Band, yoga strap, Thera-band, or any strap that is approximately fifty inches long.

What is a Core Band?

The Core Band is a specially adapted version of a resistance band. It is a canvas strip with several pockets for the placement of your hands and feet. Placing your hands inside the pockets eliminates tension in your wrists and stabilizes your shoulder girdle. You can keep your wrists straight and have the freedom to rotate your palms in many directions. Placing your feet in the pockets enhances the exercises for more core stability. Your flexibility and range of motion will determine which sleeves you use. The closer the hand placement, the more challenging the exercise will be. Start with the band in a comfortable position and try different sleeves as you become more familiar with the movements.

Core Bands are available from www.westcoastpilates.net or www.pilates.com. Alternatively, you can use a resistance band of another sort and adjust the width of your hands according to the instructions given in the exercise.

How much weight should I use?

The free weights used in this book are adjustable dumbbells and weighted balls. Start with enough weight to complete a full set of repetitions of

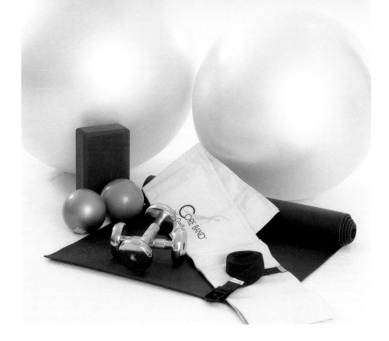

each exercise. You want to feel that you have challenged your muscles through their full range of motion, while maintaining your core alignment. Add more weight to progress. The weighted balls stabilize your wrists and create a firmer hand position for lifting with core alignment. The adjustable dumbbells are more versatile since you can add weight to the existing system without having to buy another set to progress. You can purchase free weights at any sporting goods store.

Which size stability ball should I use?

The size of the ball you choose is determined by your height. When you sit on top of the ball your feet should remain flat on the floor and your hips should be slightly higher than your knees. Stability balls generally come in three sizes and they are available all over the world from good sports stores. A common brand is Fit Ball.

Why use yoga straps and blocks?

Yoga straps and blocks aid the stretch in many of the poses. If you cannot reach your foot or the floor in the exercises, they allow you to practice the pose correctly and gently stretch your muscles. They are available at most yoga centers and fitness stores.

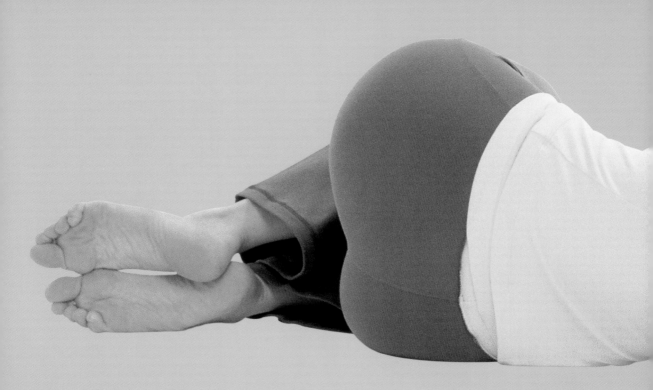

program 1

Putting the Principles to Work

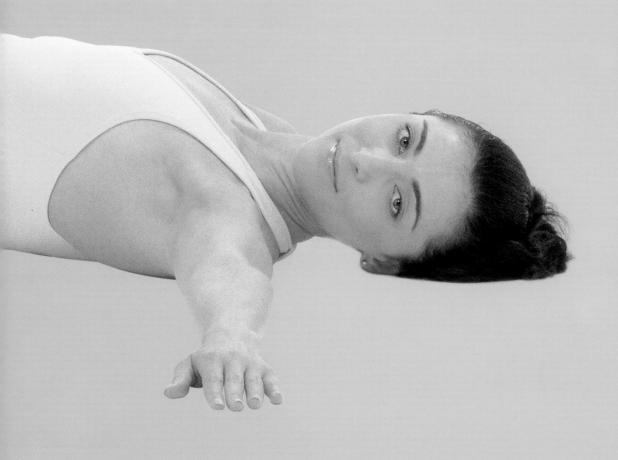

These simple but effective exercises improve strength, flexibility, balance, posture, alignment, and muscle tone. This dynamic workout will produce long, lean muscles, improve circulation and breathing, and create a sense of mental well-being.

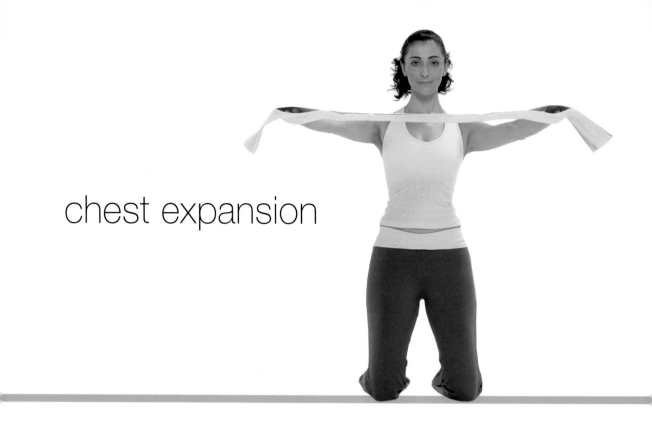

chest expansion

Benefits The flexibility and range of motion of your neck muscles affects everything from causing headaches to the alignment of your golf swing. Because the cervical spine is the most flexible part of the spine, our neck muscles must have a perfect balance of mobility and stability for correct function. Surfers, golfers, and chronic cell-phone users are experiencing a decrease in their range of motion on one side of their neck because of single-sided, repetitive use. The second benefit of this exercise comes from the very long exhalation that increases the mobility of the rib cage and re-oxygenates the body.

Starting alignment Kneel on your mat with your knees hip-distance apart. Place your hands in the sleeves next to the center pocket. Pull your band taut, lifting it to chest level. Press your shoulders down, away from your ears. Maintain your cross-point alignment from your head to your shoulders to your hips (see pages 22–23).

Movement sequence

1   Bring your arms down at the sides of your body with a long inhalation.
2   Turn your head, bringing your chin over your right shoulder.
3   Turn your head, bringing your chin over your left shoulder.
4   Turn your head to center.
5   Bring your arms up to chest level.

Repetitions Repeat the movement 5 to 10 times.

Breathing pattern Take a long inhalation as you lower your arms down at the sides of your body.

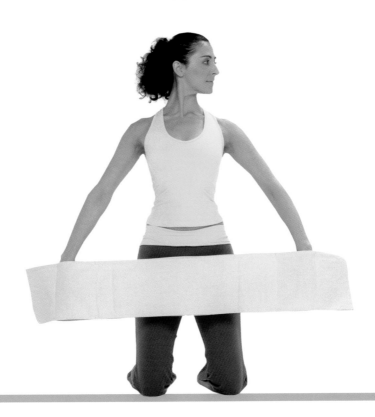

Exhale as you turn your head side to side and to the center, and continue to exhale as you lift your arms up to chest level. There are four movements to this exhalation, which allows time to fully expel the air from your lungs.

Goal Your goal is equal rotation of your head and neck. Make sure your chin does not drop down toward your shoulder as you turn. Turn only as far as you can, keeping your chin and nose parallel to the floor.

Modifications If your chin tilts, you have turned too far. Minimize your range of motion to keep the movement in alignment.

If you have difficulty kneeling, perform the exercise seated in a chair, pulling the band to your knees instead of your hips.

Take the core challenge Lower your torso and sit on your heels, keeping your arms lifted to chest level. Repeat 5 to 8 times.

Press up to the kneeling position, lower the band across your thighs, and pulse your arms back behind your torso for 20 beats.

core imprint

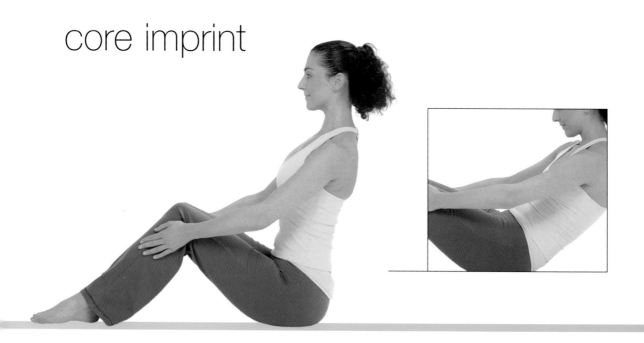

Benefits This exercise addresses the source of misalignment from your structure—the placement of the bones and, in particular, your spinal alignment. Increase your alignment through the movement of your bones in this exercise and feel your body working from the inside out.

Starting alignment Sit on your mat. Bend your knees and place your feet flat on the mat, with ankles together. Place your hands by the sides of your knees.

Movement sequence

1 Press your lower back slowly to your mat without curling your pelvis. Imagine that your hip bones are stretching away from each other and that your spine is sinking softly into your mat.

2 Release the press without tipping your hips or letting your back lift off the mat.

3 Press your shoulders to your mat, keeping the front of your rib cage still. Feel the stretch across your shoulder blades and at the front of your chest.

4 Release the press from your shoulders, keeping your shoulder blades down away from your ears and your neck relaxed.

Repetitions Do 5 presses of your lower back to the floor.

Do 5 presses of your shoulders to the floor.

Repeat the exercise, alternating the press from your lower back to your shoulders.

Breathing pattern Exhale as you press your lower back to the floor.

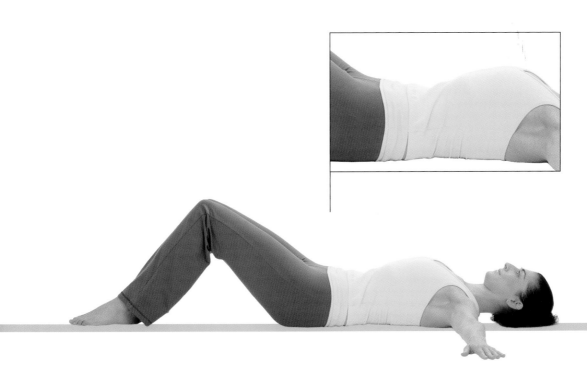

Inhale as you release your lower back. Exhale as you press your shoulders to the floor. Inhale as you release your shoulders.

Goal Your movement goal is a total release of any tension that may be preventing the imprint of your spinal alignment. The movement of this exercise is subtle. Try not to contract your muscles too much. The smaller your movement and the slower you perform it, the deeper you will work your core muscles. Also, make sure you do not arch your neck. If you find yourself doing this, correct it by gazing upward toward the ceiling, which will help keep your head in line with your spine. When you attain the full release of tension, your spine will sink into your mat with all tension totally gone.

Modification Press one hip down to the mat. Repeat with the other hip to work the sides of the body individually. Maintain an evenness of flow as you press side to side. Repeat this pattern with your shoulders.

small leg circles

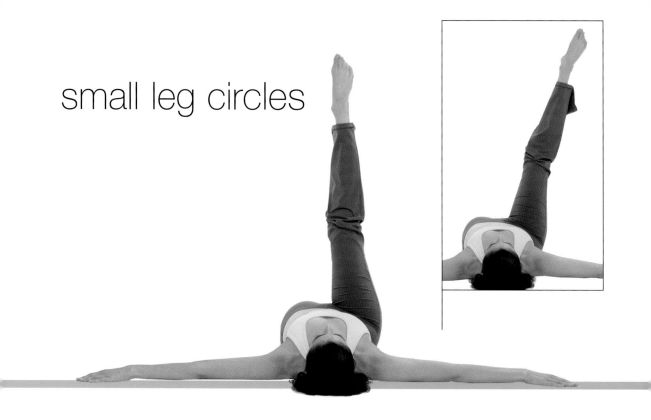

Benefits Your hips and pelvis determine the way you stand and walk. This exercise balances asymmetry in your hips and lubricates your joints.

Starting alignment Lie on your mat with your spine imprinted and your legs straight. Place your arms on the floor at the sides of your body with your palms down. Extend one leg to the ceiling at a 90-degree angle to your pelvis.

Movement sequence

1 Keep your hips completely still and make a small circle with your leg across your body and around. The smaller the circle, the deeper the movement will be in the hip joint. Circle 5 times.

2 Reverse and circle in the opposite direction 5 times.

3 Repeat with your other leg.

Repetitions Perform 1 set with each leg.

Breathing pattern Inhale and exhale with each small circle.

Goal Your goal is to keep your hip stable and unmoving as you circle your thigh bone in the hip socket. Feel how deeply you can work into the center of your joints.

Modification If you cannot straighten your leg, bend your knee to a 90-degree angle and circle with your knee bent.

Take the core challenge Increase your range of motion without releasing your hips from the floor. Anchor both hips, hold your core imprint, and circle as wide as you can, maintaining both hip and shoulder stability. Perform 5 circles in each direction before changing legs.

large leg circles

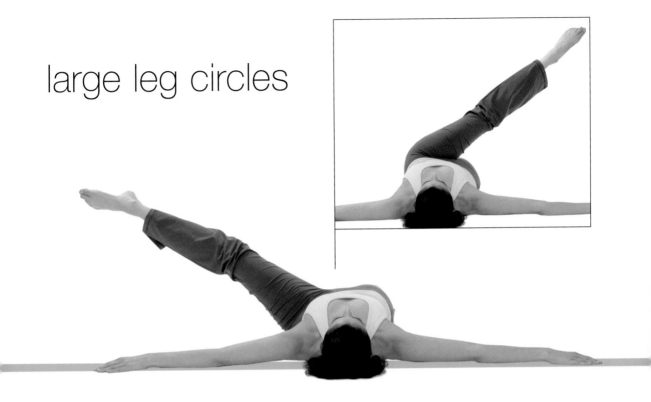

Benefits Leg circles lubricate and strengthen your hips. Keeping your hips and shoulders pressed into your mat increases the muscle work for your legs, hips, and abdominals.

Starting alignment Lie on your mat with your spine imprinted and your legs straight. Place your arms on the floor at the sides of your body with your palms down. Extend one leg to the ceiling at a 90-degree angle to your pelvis.

Movement sequence

1   With your hips and shoulders completely still, and keeping your leg straight, cross your leg over your torso.

2   Make a large, sweeping circle with your leg toward the floor and out to the other side of your body.

Repetitions Do 5 circles before repeating with your other leg.

Breathing pattern Inhale and exhale with each circle.

Goal Your goal is to circle as wide as you can while maintaining complete hip and shoulder stability.

Modification Start with a smaller range of motion and work to achieve a large, fluid circle.

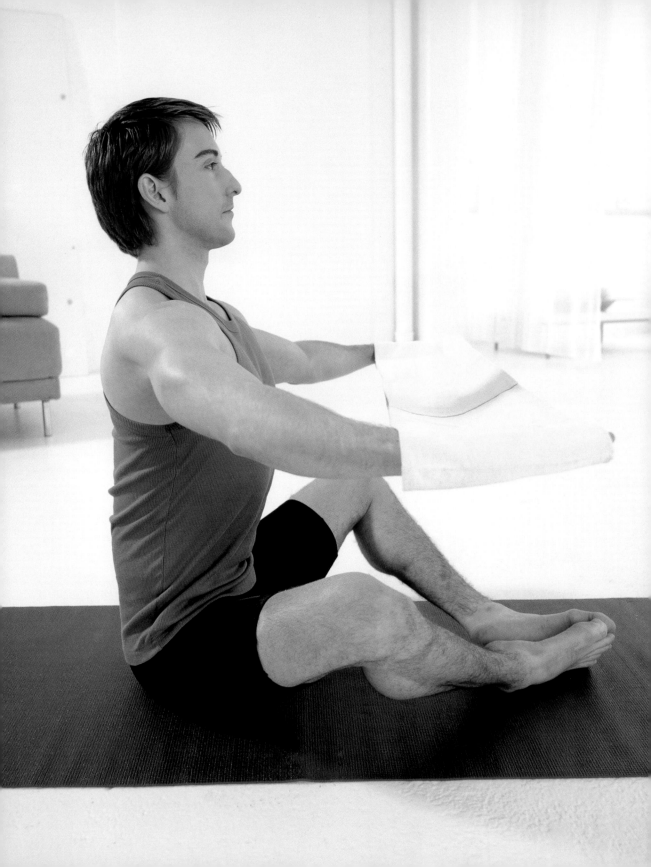

diamond contractions with taut pulls

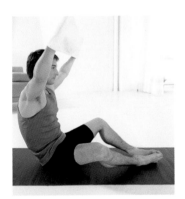

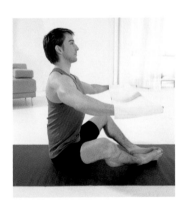

Benefits This exercise works your abdominal muscles and strengthens your arm and upper-back muscles.

Starting alignment Sit on your mat. Bring the soles of your feet together and bend your knees to form a diamond with your legs. Sit tall, lengthening your spine upward. Place your hands in the sleeves of the Core Band and lift your arms to chest level.

Movement sequence

1 Contract your abdominal muscles, rounding your back while lifting your arms over your head. Pull the band in opposition as you lift it upward.

2 Lengthen your spine from your tailbone to the back of your head. Lower the band to chest level.

Repetitions Repeat the exercise 5 times.

Breathing pattern Exhale as you contract your abdominals. Inhale as you lengthen your spine.

Goal Pull your abdominal muscles inward and hollow your abdomen as you contract. Match the deep contraction on the front of your body with a full stretch of your back muscles to release any tightness in your back. Your goal is core balance.

Modification If you feel tension in your shoulders, keep your arms at chest level as you contract.

Take the core challenge Perform the exercise with your arms overhead, pulling strongly on the band on each contraction.

cobbler's pose
Baddha Konasana

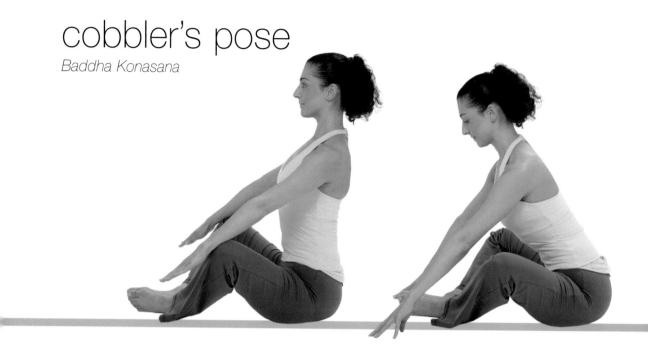

Benefits This movement releases your hips and stretches your adductors.

Starting alignment Bend your knees and place the soles of your feet together. Place your feet as close to your torso as possible without distorting your core alignment. Relax your knees and allow them to release toward the floor. Keep your arms straight.

Movement sequence

1   Gently hinge forward, keeping your back straight and your head in line with your spine. The movement should come from the pelvis.

2   Maintain openness across your back as you work slowly from the movement of your pelvis to return to your sitting position.

3   Unfold your legs and stretch them out in front of you.

Repetitions Perform the pattern once.

Breathing pattern Inhale softly and move forward on your exhalation.

It is important to draw the breath deeply into your abdomen to increase your stretch. If you feel any resistance, breathe into it to relax your muscles.

Stay in this position for 15 to 30 breaths.

Take a full breath to return to sitting.

Stretch your legs out on an exhalation.

Goal Your goal is movement from within. Focus on the release of your hip joints inside your body.

Modifications If your back rounds or your shoulders bend forward, your legs are too close to your torso. Move your feet away from your body. If you are still having difficulty, place a folded blanket or small pillow under your hips to lift your pelvis slightly.

lord of the fishes

Ardha Matsyendrasana

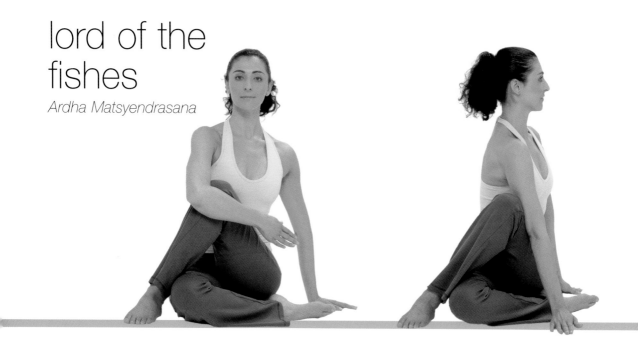

Benefits Twisting restores energy and mobility to your back. This exercise improves circulation and decreases tension in your neck and shoulders.

Starting alignment Sit on your mat with your legs extended in front of you, and place your hands on the floor at the sides of your body.

Movement sequence

1   Bend your right leg and, keeping it on your mat, bring your foot next to your left hip.
2   Cross your left foot over your right knee.
3   Lift your right arm and hold your left knee. Stretch your leg toward your chest. Keep both hips flat on your mat. Lengthen your spine upward.
4   Turn your torso to the left side. Extend your right arm and reach across your body to your right foot. Allow your head to turn with your spinal twist.

5   Release your stretch and turn to the center.
6   Unfold your legs and stretch them out in front of you.

Repetitions Go through the sequence once.

Breathing pattern Take 5 breaths to cross your legs and draw your knee to your chest.

Take 5 breaths to turn and stretch your spine.

Take 3 breaths to turn to center.

Take 1 breath to extend your legs.

Take 2 full breaths to feel the energy in your spine.

Goal Your movement goal is to keep your hips grounded and anchored to allow for greater spinal rotation. Aim for symmetry in your movements.

Modifications If you have tight hips, you may want to place a small yoga block under your hips for a more comfortable sitting position.

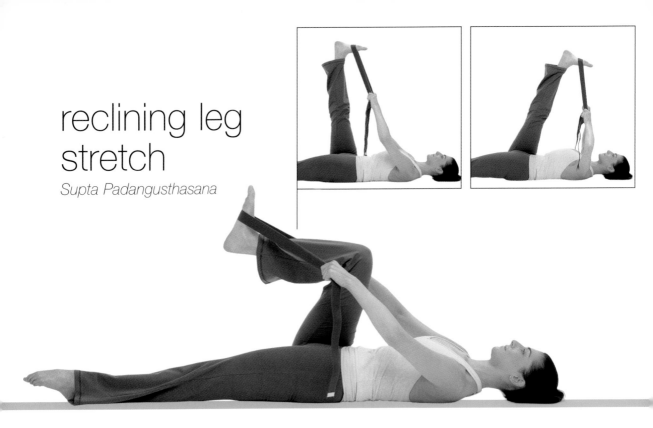

reclining leg stretch

Supta Padangusthasana

Benefits This is an excellent hamstring stretch and hip-opening exercise using a strap.

Starting alignment Lie on your mat with your legs straight and together. Align your body as if you were standing up.

Movement sequence

1 Bend one leg toward your chest. Flex your foot and place the strap around the arch of your foot.

2 Extend your leg toward the ceiling. Keep both hips pressed to your mat and the leg on the floor straight with your heel pressed to the floor.

3 Stretch your leg toward your head. Press your shoulders down to the floor for core stability.

4 Release the stretch, let go of the band, and let your leg float to the floor. Realign your body before beginning the exercise with your other leg.

Repetitions Go through the sequence once.

Breathing pattern Breathe fully as you align your torso on your mat.

Inhale as you bend your leg.

Exhale as you extend your leg toward the ceiling.

Inhale and then exhale deeply to increase the stretch of your leg.

Repeat this breath/stretch pattern 10 times.

Let your breath float with your leg as it lowers to the floor.

Goal Your goal is a complete stretch from your hip to your foot. To accomplish the stretch, your leg must be straight even if this minimizes your range of motion.

Take the core challenge Perform this exercise without the strap, holding on to your foot.

lying thigh over thigh twist

Jatara Parivartanasana (variation)

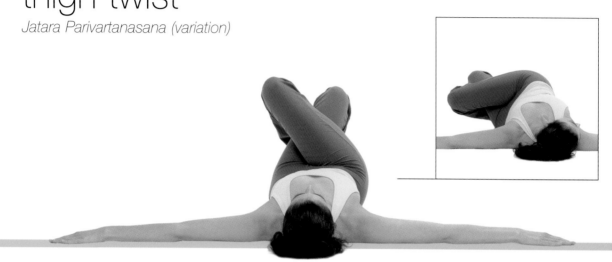

Benefits This rotational spine stretch relieves tension in the lower back, neck, and shoulders. You twist your torso more than you realize each day. This exercise helps you to unwind and relax.

Starting alignment Lie on your mat with your legs bent and feet flat. Stretch your arms out at the sides of your body with your palms facing downward.

Movement sequence

1   Lift your right leg and place it over your left thigh.

2   Roll your hips to the left, lowering your legs toward the floor. Keep both shoulders relaxed on your mat.

3   Turn your head to the right side to complete the stretch.

4   Roll your lower back and hips to your mat, bringing your legs into the center.

Repetitions Stretch once each side.

Breathing pattern Count 10 breaths on each side.

Goal Feel the spiraling of your spine from your tailbone to your head in one continuous pattern. If you feel any breaks in this line, concentrate your awareness and breathe into the release of the muscles. Work towards fluidity of your core movement.

Modifications To increase your stretch and further release tension in your back, place your opposite hand on your knee and gently press it to the floor.

basic lunge

Benefits Lunges are a great workout for the lower body. They strengthen your gluteus muscles, hamstrings, quadriceps, and calves. Make sure to use your core and keep your cross-point aligned as you lunge.

Starting alignment Stand with your feet together and hold light-to-medium hand weights.

Movement sequence

1 Take a large step forward with one leg.
2 Bend both knees so that you are in a deep lunge and your bent legs approach 90-degree angles.
3 Press off the ball of your front foot, straighten your legs, and step back to your standing position.

Repetitions Repeat 10 times, alternating legs.

Breathing pattern Exhale as you lunge. Inhale as you straighten your legs.

Goal Core stability in movement is your goal. Do not look down or lean forward but focus straight ahead to keep your shoulder placement firm as you lunge.

Make sure your spine is straight. Do not allow your front knee to press in front of your foot or you could strain your joints.

Modifications You may want to start your lunges without using hand weights. Work on your form and alignment, adding the weights as you progress.

Take the core challenge After lunging to the front, try the backward lunge. Perform the same movement, stepping to the back. Strengthen your legs by adding more repetitions. Perform 5 movements on one leg before repeating on the other. Work up to 10 repetitions on each leg and perform 3 sets to increase muscle strength.

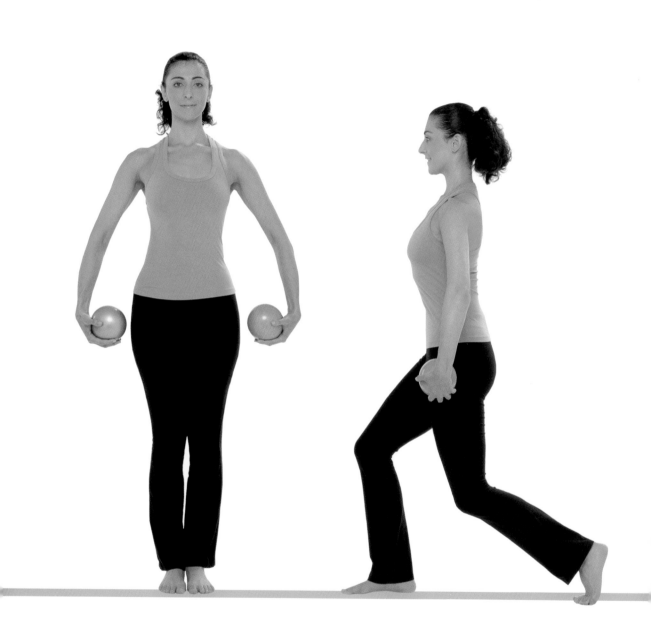

forward lunge with biceps curl

Benefits Adding the arm work to the lunges produces complete integration of concentration and your core work. Focus on your core as you initiate each movement from your center. Feel the balance of muscle work in your arms and legs. Do not lose the composition of balanced muscle work.

Starting alignment Stand with your feet together and hold light-to-medium hand weights. Your arms are at the sides of your body with your palms facing in.

Movement sequence

1 Take a large step forward with one leg.

2 Bend both knees so that you are in a deep lunge and your bent legs approach 90-degree angles. As you bend your knees, bend both arms and curl them toward your shoulders. Rotate your wrists to face your shoulders as they lift.

3 Lower your arms as you press off the ball of your foot to straighten your legs, and step back to your standing position.

Repetitions Repeat the exercise 10 times.

Breathing pattern Exhale as you lunge and curl your arms.
Inhale as you lower your arms and straighten your legs.

Goal Keep your upper arms close to your body as you lift and lower them. Make sure not to swing the weights. This is an up-and-down action, with both your arms and legs maintaining core stability. If you lean forward or use momentum, you are working out of your core, not from it.

Modifications Work with one arm at a time, using opposite arm and leg.

Take the core challenge Hold the lunge position and do 5 biceps curls before stepping back. Lunge with your other leg and repeat.

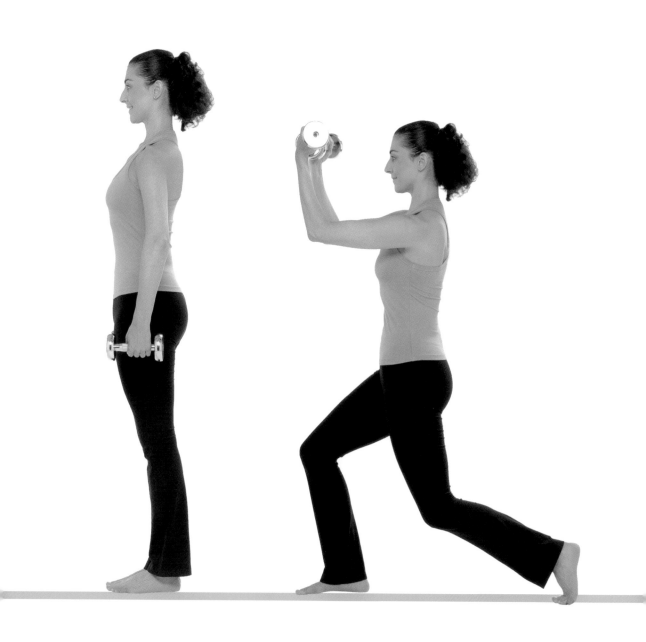

standing quadriceps bend and stretch

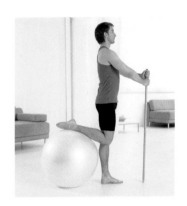

Benefits Stretching exercises help reduce muscle soreness and keep your muscles long and lean. This exercise combines strength, stretch, and balance. The stability ball increases the stretch and produces greater strength of both your working and stabilizing muscle groups.

Starting alignment Stand with your feet hip-distance apart in front of a stability ball. Hold a pole to assist your balance.

Movement sequence

1　Bend one knee and place your foot on top of the ball. Keep your hips and knees aligned.

2　Bend your standing knee, keeping your shoulder, hip, and knee alignment. Do not lean forward or move the pole. The pole should remain stable and vertical.

3　Straighten your standing leg.

4　Bend your standing knee and hold your stretch for 5 full breaths.

Repetitions Repeat the exercise 10 times. Repeat with your other leg.

Breathing pattern Inhale as you place your foot on the ball.

Exhale as you bend your knee.

Inhale as you straighten your leg.

Take 5 full breaths for your stretch.

Exhale as you lower your foot to the floor.

Goal Focus on the up-and-down movement with your chest lifted and spine straight. Maintain your cross-point alignment and move with fluidity. Do not tilt the pole or rock your torso forward.

Modifications Place your foot on a chair instead of the ball.

Take the core challenge Perform this exercise without holding the pole. Stretch your arms up in front of your torso at chest level and stay centered over your foot.

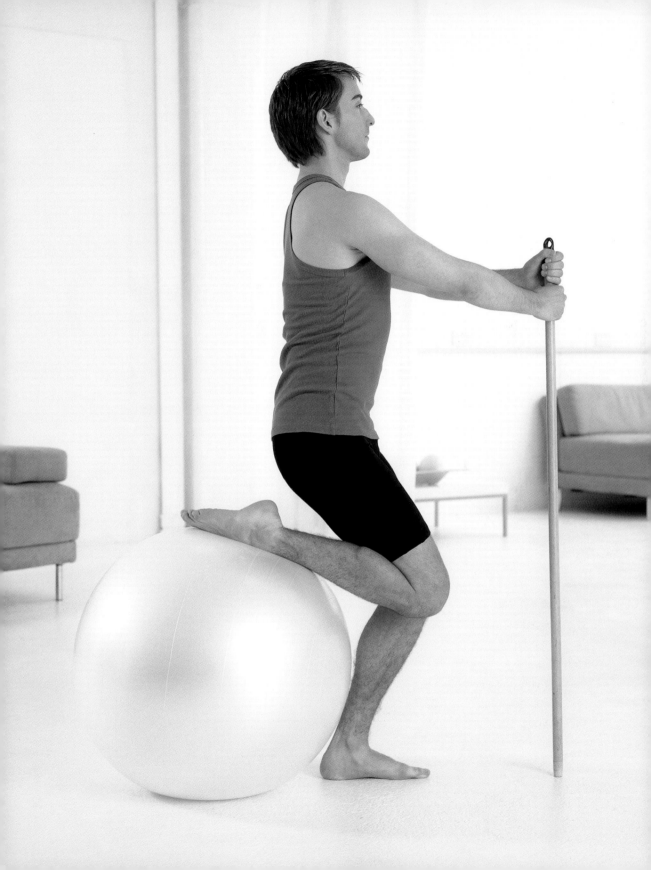

hip, thigh, and leg stretch

Benefits This movement stretches your legs, thighs, and hip flexors. It strengthens the connections from your pelvis into your legs. The hip flexors are primarily responsible for the actions of your legs as well as playing an important role in stabilizing your pelvis and lower back.

Starting alignment Stand behind your stability ball with your feet hip-distance apart.

Movement sequence

1   Lift one leg over the ball and place your foot on the floor with your knee bent. Place your hands on the ball next to your hips.

2   Stretch your other leg to straighten it out behind you with your foot flat on the floor.

3   Level your hips and press them evenly into the ball. Release the press.

4   Press your hips into the ball and stretch your back heel toward the floor, keeping your leg straight.

5   Bend your knee, releasing the stretch.

6   Release both legs and perform the exercise with the other leg.

Repetitions Press and release your hips 5 times. Stretch and release 5 times on each leg.

Breathing pattern Exhale on the hip press.

Inhale on the release.

Exhale as you press your heel down.

Inhale as you bend your knee.

Goal Try not to twist your hips. Your pelvis should remain neutral and not tip as you press down. Focus on your foot triangle as you press your heel down. Do not roll to the inside or outside of your foot. Keep your back hip and knee aligned and centered.

Modifications Perform this exercise without the ball, placing your hands on a wall for support.

Take the core challenge After doing the hip and leg stretch, lift your arms to shoulder level at the sides of your body and hinge your torso forward. Keep your spine straight and your head in line with your spine.

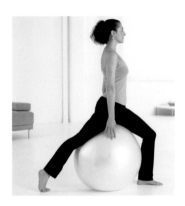

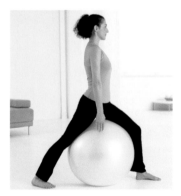

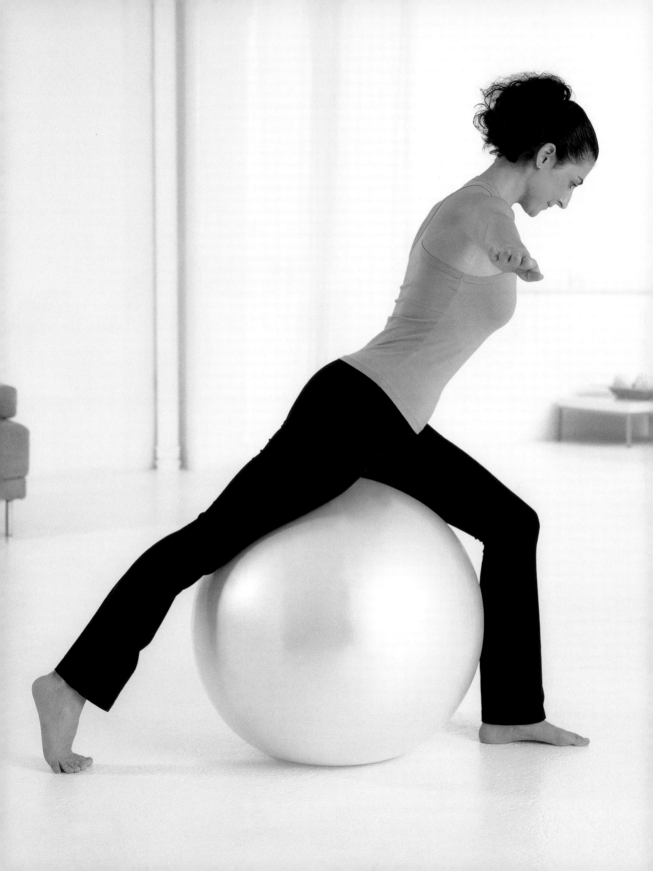

the hundred

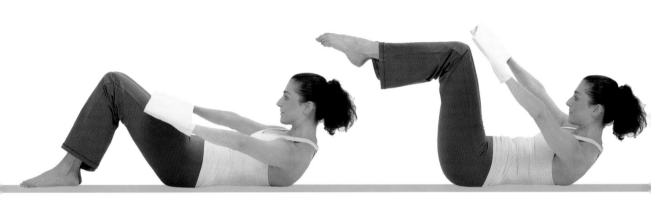

Benefits The Hundred is the ultimate core exercise because it stimulates circulation, improves breathing, and strengthens your deepest core muscles. The Hundred with the Core Band works the body in opposition because the core remains solid as your arms and legs stretch in opposite directions.

Starting alignment Lie on your mat on your back. Bend your knees and place your feet on your mat. Bring your toes, ankles, and knees together. Place your hands in the sleeves of the Core Band, keeping your wrists straight. Pull the band in opposition and keep it pulled taut through the exercise.

Movement sequence

1   Lift your upper body off the mat and reach your arms toward your knees, pulling your shoulder blades down and together.

2   Using a strong and deep contraction, pulse your upper body and band toward your legs. Match your breath to your movements, breathing in for 5 inhalations and breathing out for 5 exhalations. Stay in this position for 20 counts.

3   Slowly lift your legs off the floor to a 90-degree angle. Continue the pulsing movements, reaching your upper body and band toward your knees while you continue the breathing pattern for 20 more counts.

4   Slowly extend your legs to the ceiling and keep pulsing toward your toes for the next 20 counts.

5   Reach your arms over your head, using the pulsing movement and breath pattern for an additional 20 counts.

6   Begin to lower your legs on a diagonal away from

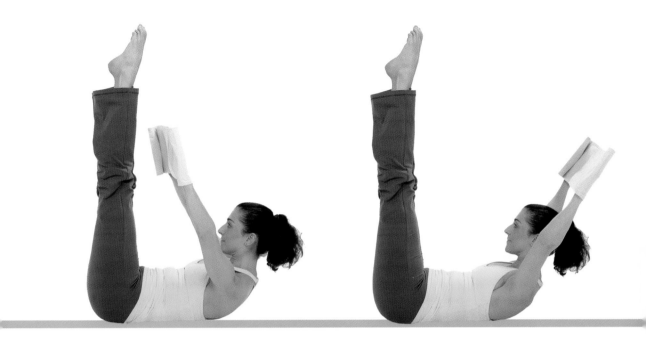

your torso as you continue to pulse your arms over your head. Lower your legs as close to the ground as possible without allowing your spine to lift from the mat and complete The Hundred with your last set of 20. Lower your head to the mat. Release your arms down, bend your knees, and place your feet on the mat.

Repetitions One time through this movement pattern is enough to tone your deep abdominal muscles.

Breathing pattern Inhale for 5 counts, matching the beats of your arms, and exhale with 5 inhalations and 5 exhalations. If this is too difficult at first, use a pattern of 2 inhalations and 3 exhalations. Take a full breath to lower your upper body and place your feet on the mat.

Goal Your movement goal is core stabilization while expanding and contracting the rib cage. Your abdominal muscles must stay scooped and your back must remain flat on the floor as you stretch your arms overhead and lower your legs. Feel your back flat on your mat throughout the exercise. Feel your shoulders pulling down and keep your abdominal muscles engaged.

Modifications You may need to keep your knees bent to maintain your spinal alignment and keep your back pressed to the floor. Decrease the number of repetitions if you feel any tension in your neck or any discomfort in your lower back. As you progress, make sure the transition to the next position is performed with precision, and never allow your back to lift from the mat.

rolling like a ball

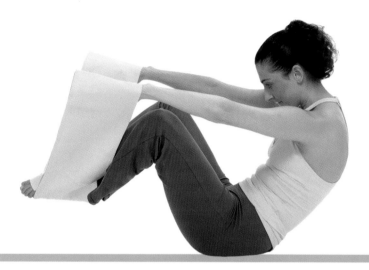

Benefits The articulation of your spine through the rolling movement of this exercise restores the natural alignment of your spine. The Core Band helps you to maintain your rounded shape, ensuring that you roll smoothly and place each vertebra on your mat like the spokes of a wheel. This exercise is restorative as it massages your spine.

Starting alignment Sit on your mat. Place your feet in the center pocket of the band and place your hands in the sleeves next to the ends of the band. Bend your knees to your chest. Lift your legs off your mat and open your knees until they are shoulder-distance apart. Keep your feet together. Strongly contract your abdominal muscles and round your back. Bring your head toward your knees to follow the roundness of your spine.

Movement sequence

1   Maintaining your body design, roll back to your mat, rolling like a ball and touching each vertebra to your mat, very slowly and with controlled precision.

2   Roll only to your shoulder blades; never onto your neck. Roll up to the sitting position, keeping your back rounded.

Repetitions Repeat the exercise 5 times.

Breathing pattern Inhale as you roll back. Exhale as you roll up.

Goal Feel each vertebra stretch to the mat to increase your spinal mobility. This exercise helps lengthen and massage your spine. Your goal is the complete control of your movement from the core contraction of your abdominal muscles. Avoid

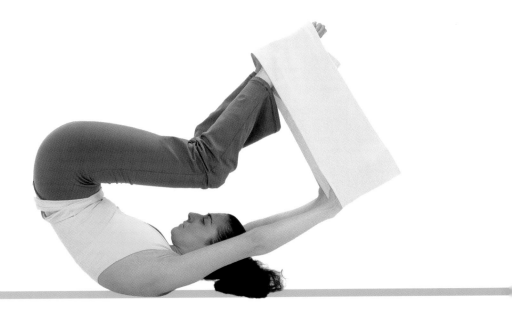

heaving your body up and down by yanking your legs. This is all about control.

Modification If you have difficulty rolling with your feet in the band, place the band under your calves.

To perform this exercise without the band, place your hands on the outside of your ankles. Keep your rolling movements controlled. Never use your body's momentum or you will miss the full value of the core work.

Take the core challenge For a more challenging position, place your hands in the sleeves next to your feet. Place your hands on your shins and roll without changing the distance from your shoulders to your knees.

single leg stretch

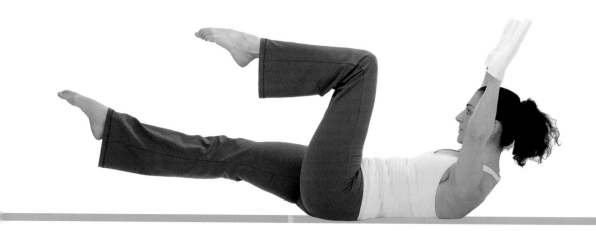

Benefits The principles of working in opposition, imprinting the spine through flexion and extension, and matching breath to movement are all challenged in this movement.

Starting alignment Lie on your mat with your spine imprinted and your legs straight. Place your hands in the sleeves of the Core Band with your arms slightly wider than your shoulders. Bend one knee and bring your leg toward your chest. Lift your upper back and head and reach your band toward your feet.

Movement sequence

1   Lift your extended leg off the mat to hip level. Keep your spine imprinted.

2   Press your knee toward your shoulder while contracting your upper abdominal muscles and reaching your shoulders to your knee.

3   Extend your leg out, switching the positions of your legs, and extend your arms overhead.

Repetitions Repeat the exercise 10 times, alternating legs.

Breathing pattern Inhale as you stretch your band to your knee.
Exhale as you extend your arms overhead.

Goal Feel your abdominal muscles pressed to your spine and your spine imprinted on your mat. Feel the extension of your leg away from your torso without kicking your leg out.

Modifications If you cannot keep your spine flat on your mat, lift your legs toward the ceiling.

Take the core challenge The lower your legs are to your mat, the more difficult it will be to maintain the imprint of your spine.

double leg stretch

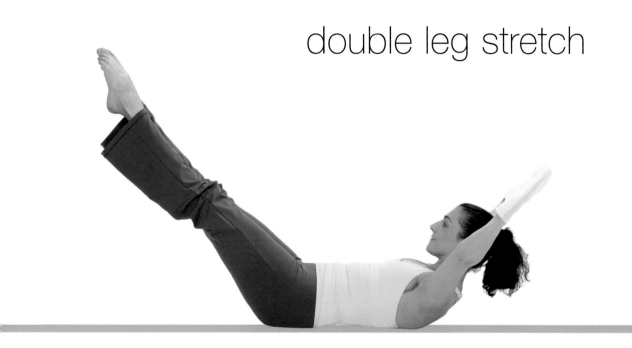

Benefits You can achieve ultimate core stability by extending both arms and legs away from your torso while anchoring your shoulders and hips to your mat.

Starting alignment Lie on your mat with your spine imprinted and your legs straight. Place your hands in the sleeves of the Core Band with your arms slightly wider than your shoulders. Bend your knees and bring your legs toward your chest. Lift your upper back and head and reach your band toward your feet. Keep your spine imprinted.

Movement sequence

1   Bend your knees toward your chest and shoulders while contracting your upper abdominal muscles and reaching your arms toward your knee with 2 small pulses.

2   Extend your legs out in a diagonal line. At the same time, lift your arms past your ears.

Repetitions Repeat the exercise 10 times.

Breathing pattern Inhale twice as you stretch your band to your knee.

Exhale as you extend your arms overhead.

Goal Your movement goal is to extend your arms and legs low to the ground without releasing your core alignment. Lengthen fully from your fingertips to your toes as if you are being pulled in opposite directions.

Modification Extend your legs toward the ceiling to maintain your imprinted spine position.

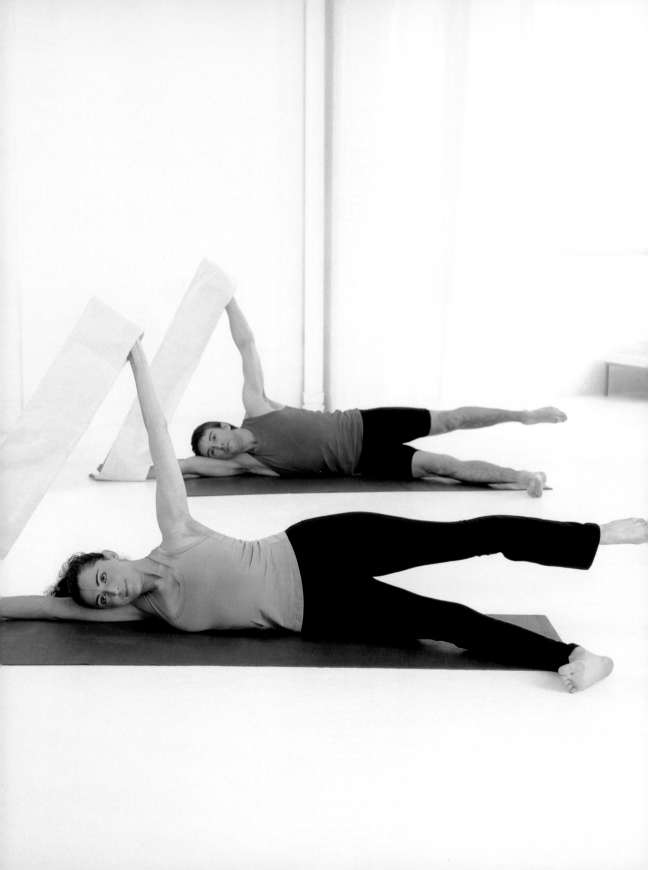

side kick series

Benefits This series of four exercises is designed to stretch, tone, and lengthen the leg muscles simultaneously. The exercises work to increase hip mobility and tone the hip muscles. Perform these exercises sequentially before repeating them with the other leg.

Starting alignment Lie on the back edge of your mat on the side of your body. Form a straight line with your back and your hips, placing shoulder over shoulder and hip over hip. Stretch your lower arm out on the floor and rest your head on it. Place your hands in the sleeves of your Core Band. Extend your top arm up, pressing your band over your head toward the ceiling. Bring your feet to the front edge of your mat, creating a slight angle to your body. Keep your shoulders and your hips aligned and stable throughout the exercise.

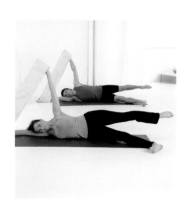

Movement sequence: Point Up/Flex Down

1   Point your foot and lift your top leg as high as you can without rolling your hip or leg forward or back. Keep your foot parallel to the floor as you lift your leg. Point your foot as you lift.

2   Flex your foot and lower your leg on top of your other leg, stretching your leg from your hip so it reaches out of your hip and past your foot on the mat. Flex your foot as you lower.

Repetitions Repeat the exercise 10 times.

Breathing pattern Inhale as you lift your leg.

Exhale as you lower your leg.

Movement sequence: Pulse to Sweep

1   Lift your top leg a few inches so it is level with your hip and parallel to the floor.

2   Sweep your leg in front of you, as far as you can without swaying your band over your head. Pulse your leg in front of your body twice.

3   Sweep your leg backward, keeping it hip distance above your mat.

Repetitions Repeat the exercise 10 times.

Breathing pattern Inhale twice as you pulse your leg.

Exhale as you sweep back.

side kick series continued

Movement sequence: Bicycle

1 Bend your top knee in front of your body at hip level. Make sure your leg is parallel to the floor.

2 Extend your leg in front of your body, stretching it out from your hip to your toes, keeping it at hip level.

3 Sweep your leg back as far as possible, maintaining your core stability and keeping your leg parallel to the floor. Hold your leg back, stretching from your hip to your toes.

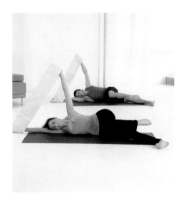

4 Bend your leg and stretch it to the front of your body to begin again.

5 Reverse the exercise by holding your leg in the back position and sweeping forward.

Repetitions Pedal forward 5 times and pedal backward 5 times.

Breathing pattern Each cycle of your leg should take two full breaths.

Movement sequence: Leg Beats

1 Lift your top leg as far as you can without twisting your knee upward or changing your hip alignment. Stretch your leg behind your torso and keep your legs straight.

2 Point your foot and beat your leg toward the floor with four small, sharp movements.

3 Flex your foot and repeat the four beats.

Repetitions Alternate the point and flex movements and perform 5 sets of each foot position.

Breathing pattern Inhale twice and exhale twice with each small beat.

Goal This entire series is performed by engaging your core muscles to stabilize your trunk as you work from your shoulders and hips to your legs. Use precise movements initiated from your core. If your top arm moves, you have lost your core alignment.

Modifications Lower your top arm and place your hand on your mat in front of your chest for balance.

Take the core challenge Lift your head up and keep it in line with your spine through the series.

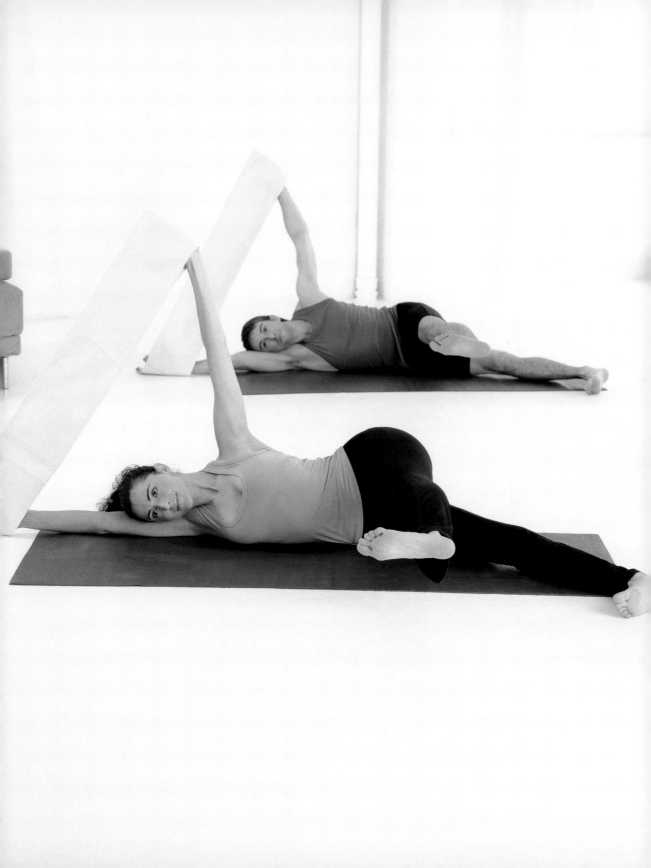

reclined twist

Jarthara Parivartanasana

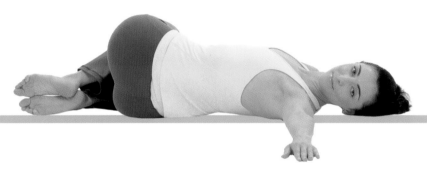

Benefits This pose releases tension from your lower back, waist, and chest. It improves circulation and alleviates both mental and physical stress.

Starting alignment Lie on your back with your knees bent and feet flat on your mat. Extend your arms out at the sides of your body with your palms down.

Movement sequence

1　Bring your knees toward your chest, allowing your lower back to release into your mat.

2　Lower your legs to one side of your body, placing them on the floor. Let go of any tension you may feel. Focus your attention on the stretch from your pelvis to your chest and shoulders.

3　Gently turn your head in the opposite direction from your legs.

4　Roll your knees into the center position.

5　Repeat the movement to the other side.

Repetitions Perform this once on each side.

Breathing pattern Inhale as you lift your knees to your chest.

Fully exhale as you lower your knees to the side.

Take 3 full breaths in this position.

Inhale and exhale to return to the center.

Goal Your movement goal is to keep your shoulders down to increase the stretch across your shoulders and chest. With each exhalation, allow the weight of your legs to draw out your body's tension.

Modifications You may find it more comfortable to place a folded blanket under your knees.

seated twist

Bharadvajasana

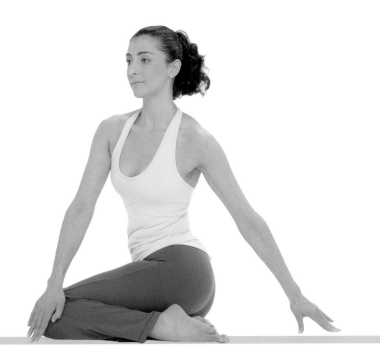

Benefits This exercise unwinds mind and body. It improves breathing, opens your chest, and refreshes the spirit.

Starting alignment Sit with your knees bent to the left side of your body and tuck your feet close to your right hip. Place your right foot into the arch of your left foot. Lengthen your spine and sit up tall.

Movement sequence

1   Turn your torso to the left.
2   Reach across your body with your right arm and place it on your left knee.
3   Stretch your left arm behind you and place it on the floor.
4   Untwist into the center position.

Repetitions Repeat the exercise 3 times before changing directions.

Breathing pattern Inhale and exhale as you twist. Stay in the twist for 3 full breaths. Use a full breath to turn to center.

Goal Keep your hips and shoulders level as you twist. Your head turns with the twist of your spine. Anchor your right thigh to your mat and try not to lean to the right side. Do not release your rib cage or arch your upper back.

Modifications Twist only as far as you can while maintaining your core alignment.

Take the core challenge When you twist to the left side, lift your left arm and stretch it across your back to touch your right arm. Place it on the floor. Repeat this movement 3 times.

head to knee pose

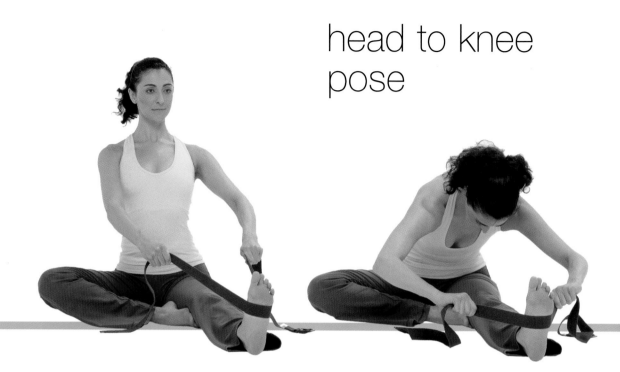

Benefits This forward stretch opens the chest and stretches your lower back, hamstrings, and calves all at once. Forward-bending movements aid spinal elasticity and joint mobility. Using a yoga strap helps as you begin with this stretch.

Starting alignment Sit on your mat with your legs straight in front of you and your spine straight. Hold your strap in your hands.

Movement sequence

1 Bend one leg and place your foot on your other thigh as close to your hip as is comfortable. Relax your bent knee to the floor.

2 Place your strap around your extended foot and flex your foot.

3 Lengthen your spine and stretch upward, keeping your leg straight.

4 With your back straight, hinge forward from your hips and stretch your torso toward your leg.

5 Begin to round over your leg, starting from your pelvis to your lower back to your upper back and head.

6 Round your back up fluidly to return to your sitting position.

Repetitions Do 1 pattern on each side.

Breathing pattern Inhale and exhale to prepare for the stretch.

Take 3 breaths in the hinge stretch.

Inhale and exhale 5 times as you stretch over your legs.

Take a full breath to release.

Goal Keep your extended leg straight, but be careful not to lock your knee. Concentrate on stretching out

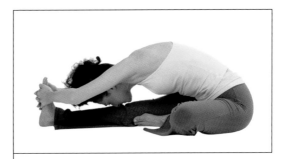

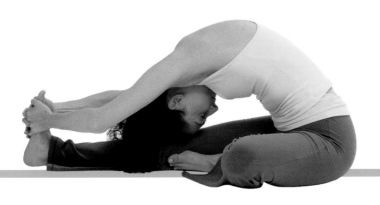

and over rather than pulling down. Initiate your stretch from your hips and pelvis and do not collapse your torso to your leg. Do not allow your extended leg to roll out. Keep your knee and foot facing the ceiling. Stretch from your core. Do not pull with your arms. Relax and allow your spine to stretch fully. Release any resistance you might feel.

Modifications Sit on a rolled blanket to assure the stretch is being initiated from your hips and legs, not from your lower back.

Take the core challenge Use your arms instead of the strap to stretch over your leg. Hold your wrists around your foot for a deeper stretch. To increase the stretch still further, try to place your nose to your extended leg, so that you're sitting as flat against your extended leg as possible.

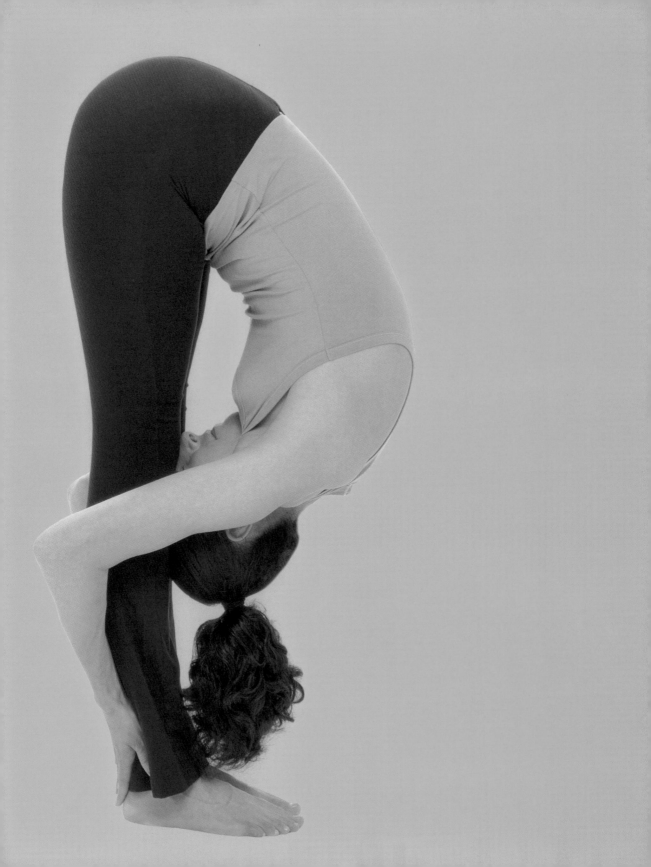

program 2

Dynamic Strength Conditioning

This workout focuses on core conditioning by bringing together an innovative blend of fitness regimens. With this program you will engage all the muscle groups essential for conditioning the core, including the hip, abdominal, leg, and back muscles. The focus is on integrating, rather than isolating, your muscle work.

mountain pose
Tadasana

Benefits This pose is the foundation for all yoga standing poses. It improves posture, alignment, and balance. Use this pose whenever you need to feel centered.

Alignment

1   Check your foot alignment by making sure that your foot center at the front of your foot triangle is in alignment with your heel and ankle.

2   Bring your thighs and hips in line, placing your hips over your ankles.

3   Lengthen your torso and press your shoulders lightly down, lifting your chest.

4   Keep your gaze straight ahead.

5   Feel the plumb line of your body from the top of your head through the center of your chest through your pelvis and down to your feet.

Breathing pattern Take 10 breaths and focus on standing in a balanced position of strength.

Goal Maintaining this alignment will improve your posture. Make sure not to tuck your pelvis or arch your lower back.

Modifications If you feel unstable with your feet together, stand with your feet hip-distance apart.

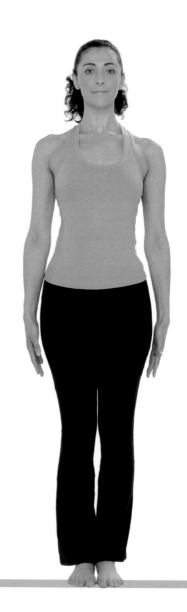

tree pose

Vrksasana

Benefits This pose strengthens your feet, and improves balance and focus.

Starting alignment Stand in Mountain Pose (see opposite).

Movement sequence

1. Bend one knee, lift your foot, and place it on the center of your other thigh with your toes pointing down. Stretch out at the side of your body, opening from your hip. Keep your pelvis level.

2. Hold your arms diagonally out to the side or leave them over your head, with your palms pressed together.

3. Lower your leg to Mountain Pose.

4. Repeat with your other leg.

Repetitions Perform this pose once on each side.

Breathing pattern Exhale as you lift your leg. Inhale as you lift your arms.

Take 5 full breaths before lowering your leg.

Goal Do not let your hip lift as you lift your leg. Open your hip so your knee is at the side of your body. Keep your sternum level and your shoulders relaxed.

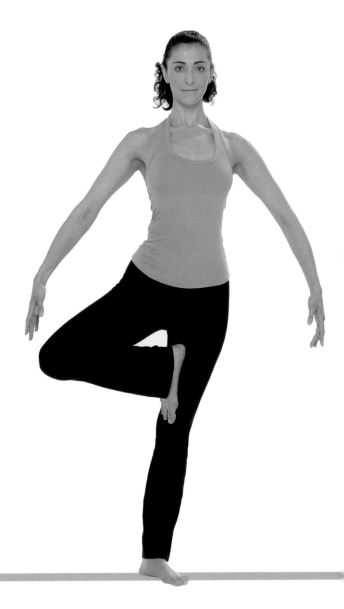

standing forward bend

Uttanasana

Benefits This pose stretches your lower back, hamstrings, and calves. Concentrate on the release of the spine and neck. It calms and quiets your mind and produces an all-over sense of well-being. This simple stretch can be added to the beginning or the end of your program or done any time your body feels tight from being in one position for a long time.

Starting alignment Stand with your feet together or, if you find it easier, hip-distance apart. Relax your arms at the sides of your body.

Movement sequence

1 Stretch your torso forward from your hips, reaching over your thighs.

2 Place your hands on the floor in front of your feet in line with your toes.

3 Stay balanced and grounded into your feet. Keep your spine long and fluid as you return to your standing position.

Repetition Perform this pose once.

Breathing pattern Exhale to bend forward. Take 5 soft breaths to stretch to your legs. Inhale to come to standing.

Goal Keep your abdomen concave, as if there is a breath of space between it and your thighs. Let the tension release from your body. Do not lean forward into your hands or press back on your heels. The balance and counterbalance of the stretch comes from your torso and hips. Keep your hips over your heels and your head in line with your spine.

Modifications You may want to begin this pose by placing a block in front of your feet. Stretch forward and place your hands on the block. The block should be directly under your shoulders.

Take the core challenge Place your arms around the backs of your calves and try to get your head as close to your knees as possible without having to bend your knees.

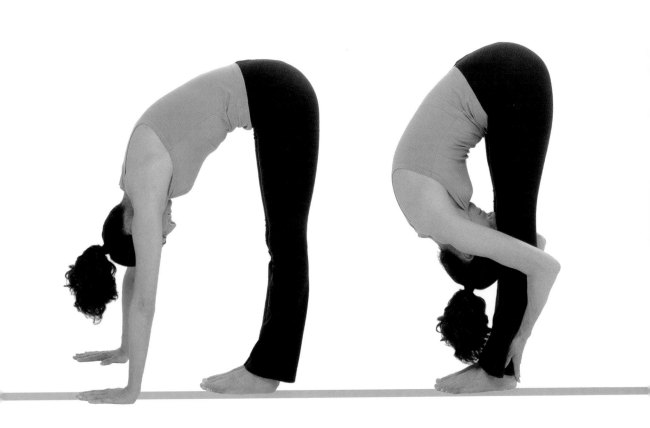

triangle pose 1
Trikonasana

Benefits This pose stretches your legs, opens your hips, and tones your oblique and back muscles.

Starting alignment Stand with your feet wide apart.

Movement sequence

1 Extend your arms out at the sides of your body.

2 Turn your right foot in. Turn your left leg and foot out directly to the side of your body.

3 Stretch your body to the left side as far as you can without leaning forward, and place your left hand on your left leg.

4 Lift your right arm directly to the ceiling, stretching upward through your chest, lengthening your spine, and gazing at your upper hand.

5 Turn your head to look straight again. Engage your muscles from the ground upward and return to your standing position.

Repetitions Perform this pose once on each side.

Breathing pattern Inhale as you lift your arms.

Exhale as you stretch over.

Take 3 full breaths in the pose.

Lift your torso up with an inhalation.

Goal Make sure your movement comes from your hips and do not allow your shoulders to round forward.

Take the core challenge Place your hand on the floor behind your foot.

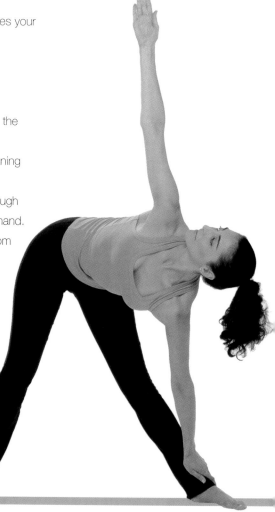

triangle pose 2
Utthita Parsvakonasana

Benefits This pose increases hip and hamstring flexibility.

Starting alignment Stand with your feet wide apart.

Movement sequence

1   Extend your arms out to your sides.
2   Turn your right foot in. Turn your left leg and foot out directly to the side of your body.
3   Bend your left knee and lunge deeply to the side.
4   Lengthen your spine upward. Stretch your body to the left side as far as you can without leaning forward, and place your left hand on your left leg or foot.
5   Lift your right arm directly to the ceiling, stretching upward through your chest, lengthening your spine, and gazing at your upper hand.
6   Turn your head to look straight ahead. Engage your muscles from the ground upward and return to your standing position.

Repetitions Perform this exercise once on each side.

Breathing pattern Inhale as you lift your arms.

Exhale as you stretch over.

Take 3 full breaths in the pose.

Lift your torso up with an inhalation.

Goal Make sure your movement comes from your hips and do not allow your shoulders to round forward.

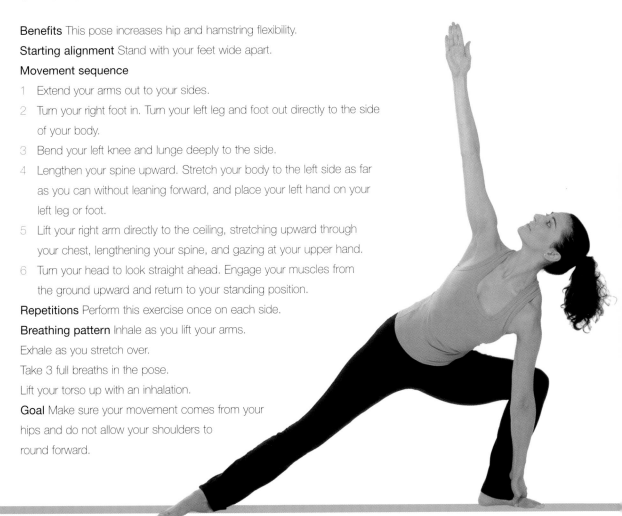

standing side bend

Benefits This beautiful stretch tones your waistline and works your obliques. The depth of your movement will depend on your core flexibility and will progress with your practice of this exercise.

Starting alignment Stand with your heels together and your toes apart, as in ballet first position. Plant your feet firmly into the ground and do not lock your knees.

Movement sequence

1   Lift your arms up over your head and press your palms together. Keep your arms straight.
2   Lengthen your torso upward, stretching from your hips to your rib cage.
3   Reach over to the side of your body, bending at your waist and keeping both hips facing forward.
4   Stretch to the opposite wall, not to the floor.
5   Stretch up to your standing position before repeating the movement to the other side.

Repetitions Repeat 3 times, alternating sides.

Breathing pattern Inhale as you lift your arms. Exhale as you stretch to the side.

Inhale and then, as you exhale, stretch further to the side.

Take 2 more breaths, stretching further with each exhalation.

Inhale and exhale to lift your torso to the center.

Goal Your movement goal is to stretch to the side without turning your hips or shoulders. Do not let your shoulders raise upward or roll forward. Keep your head in line with your spine. Keep your arms centered around your ears and do not hold your breath. All side bends should be performed by first lengthening your torso upward out of your hips before beginning the side movement. This will prevent sinking into your hips, which lessens the amount of stretch you will be able to accomplish as you reach to the side.

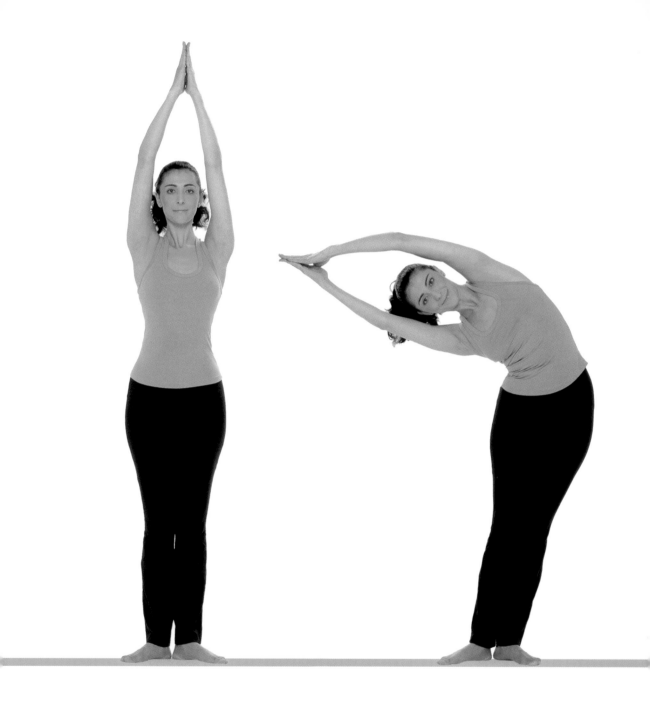

neck and shoulder stretch

Benefits People with generally good posture can tend to lose correct spinal alignment at their shoulder level. Remember, your spine does not end at your neck or even at the base of your skull but continues up to the level of your nose. Allowing your head to jut forward increases the compression in your cervical spine and decreases blood flow into the head. This exercise helps correct poor upper-spine posture.

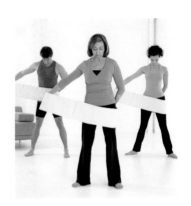

Starting alignment Stand with your feet hip-distance apart. Place your hands in the sleeves of your Core Band. Relax your arms down at the sides of your body. Make sure you place your shoulders directly over your hips and do not hunch forward as you begin the exercise.

Movement sequence

1   Place one hand on your thigh. Lift the other arm up at the side of your body. Lower your head as you bring your chin to your chest.

2   Circle your head over your shoulder, bringing your chin parallel to the floor while pressing your opposite shoulder down.

3   Pulse your head over your shoulder with 10 small pulses.

4   Bring your chin to your chest.

Repetitions Repeat the pattern 3 times on each side.

Breathing pattern Inhale as you bring your chin to your chest.

Exhale as you circle your head over your shoulder.

Inhale twice and exhale twice as you pulse your head over your shoulder.

Use a full breath to circle to the other side and to complete the exercise.

Goal Your goal is to improve and equalize the length, muscle tone, and symmetry of your neck muscles.

Modifications Perform the movement without the band while you are sitting at your desk or after a long conversation on the telephone.

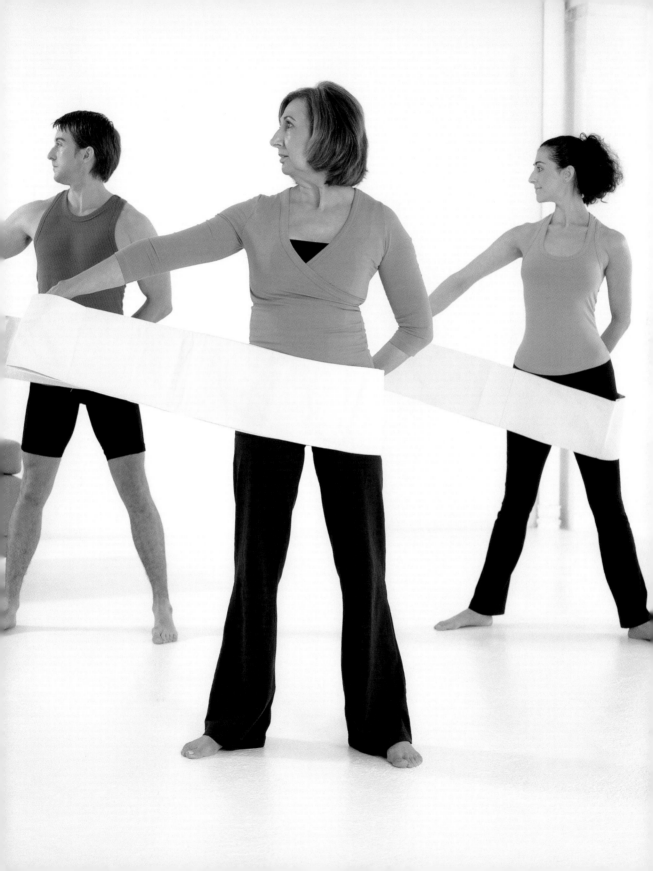

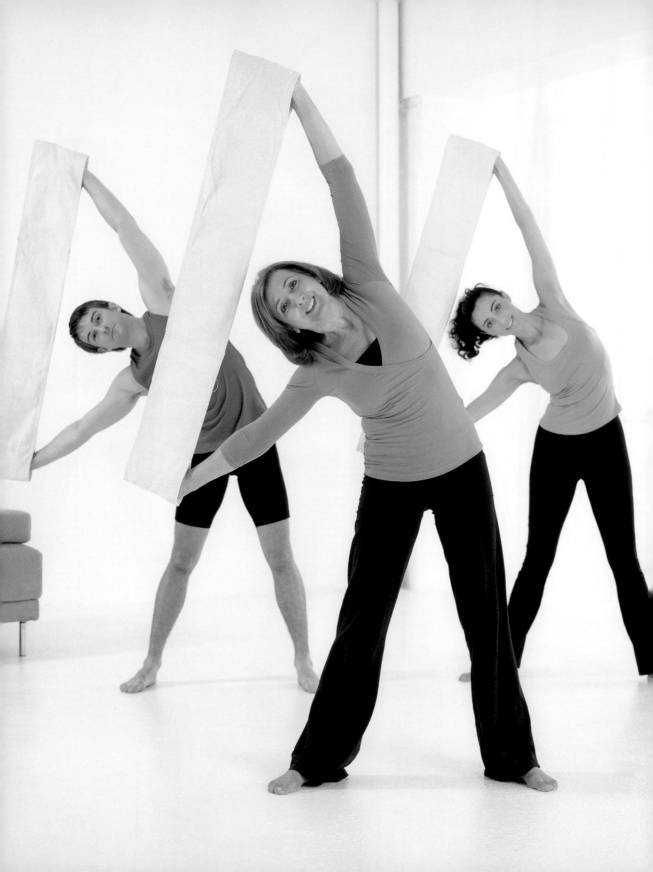

side stretch with cross reach

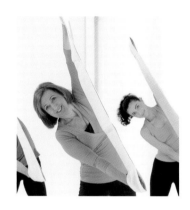

Benefits Most of your daily activities are one sided, causing one side of your body to be dominant. This exercise is designed to rebalance both sides of your core muscles.

Starting alignment Stand with your feet apart. Place your hands in the sleeves of the Core Band. Bring your arms over your head, pulling your band taut.

Movement sequence

1. Stretch your upper body over to the side, keeping your shoulders and your hips in a straight line.
2. Reach your bottom hand across your body. Keep your shoulders in alignment and your head in line with your spine.
3. Sweep your arm back to the side of your body. Repeat the arm movement 5 times.
4. Stretch the band away from your torso as if you are pushing it away from you. Release the stretch. Repeat this stretch 5 times.
5. Pull your band taut and raise your torso to the standing position.

Repetitions Repeat the pattern 4 times, alternating sides.

Breathing pattern Inhale and exhale as you stretch to the side, taking 2 full breaths to stretch.

Inhale as you reach your arm across your body.

Exhale as you sweep back.

Inhale into the stretch as you push away.

Exhale as you release.

Inhale and exhale as you lift your torso up to the center.

Goal Stabilize your shoulders and hips to get the utmost work in your body. If you feel any discomfort in your back or your knees, your shoulder and hips have rotated. Stretch only as far as you can while maintaining core postural alignment.

standing roll-down

Benefits This exercise aligns all your core muscles. You may want to end your workout with this movement or do it whenever you feel a need for physical and/or mental realignment.

Starting alignment Stand with your feet hip-distance apart. Distribute your body weight evenly into your foot triangles. Center your joints and align your hips and shoulders. Place your head in line with your spine.

Movement sequence

1 Lift your arms overhead.

2 Begin to lower your arms toward the floor, followed by your head, neck, and shoulders.

3 Continue to roll down, stretching your spine and peeling each vertebra as if you were stretching away from an imaginary wall. Keep your tailbone reaching down to the floor and your abdominal muscles pulled inward with your navel-to-spine contraction. Draw your shoulders down, away from your ears, and roll as far as you can, keeping your core alignment.

4 Begin to roll up, slowly. Visualize placing each vertebra against an imaginary wall.

Repetitions Repeat the exercise 3 times.

Breathing pattern Take 4 long, full breaths to roll down.

Inhale and exhale when you have reached your full stretch over.

Take 4 long, full breaths to roll up.

Goal Your goal is to maintain your postural alignment through activity and create healthy muscular patterns.

Modifications Perform this exercise against the wall. Stand with your feet about 10 inches away from the wall. Press your back and shoulders against it. Roll your torso down one vertebra at a time. Visualize that you are rounding over a giant ball. Keep your tailbone pressed into the wall. Slowly roll up, lengthening your spine and working deeply from your core muscles.

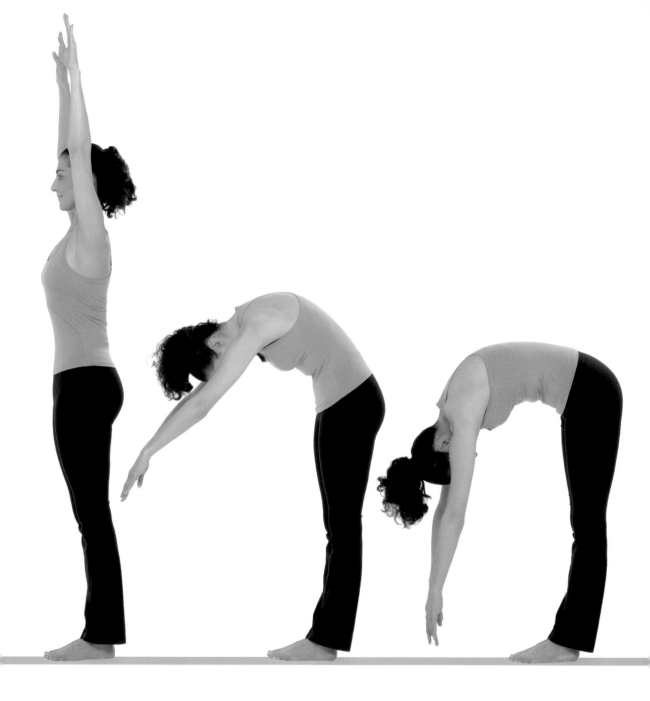

the saw

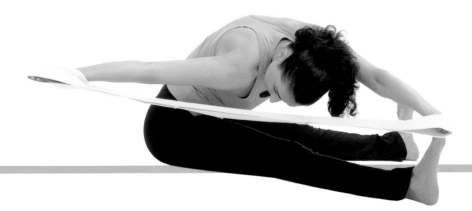

Benefits The Saw is a rotational stretch that works your waist and back muscles. It also stretches your hamstrings and releases stress in your lower back.

Starting alignment Sit on your mat with your legs in a wide V. Place your hands in the sleeves of the Core Band and pull it taut.

Movement sequence

1   Lift your band over your head.

2   Point your feet and stretch across your body, reaching your arm past the opposite foot. Keep both hips anchored to your mat.

3   Reach past your toes on the outside of your foot and stretch forward, sliding your hand in a "sawing" motion. Pull your band back by reaching your opposing shoulder and arm to the back of the room, working in opposition. Saw past your toes 10 times.

4   Round your back to sit up and lift your arms over your head. Repeat the exercise on the other side.

Repetitions Repeat the exercise 2 times.

Breathing pattern Inhale as you lift your band overhead.

Exhale as you stretch across your body.

Inhale twice and exhale twice with your sawing motion.

Take a full breath to round your back up.

Goal Keep both hips pressed to your mat and your abdominal muscles pulled inward and upward. Make sure your head follows the line of your spine.

Modifications If you have difficulty sitting tall with your legs straight, bend one leg. Stretch over the straight leg and gradually straighten your bent knee.

open leg rocker

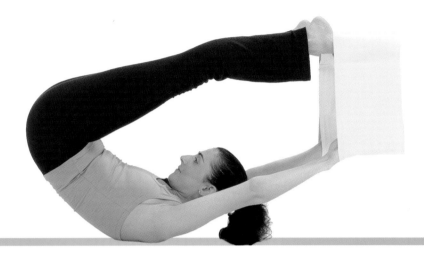

Benefits This exercise helps build a strong, stable core, working your abdominals and back muscles.

Starting alignment Sit on your mat. Bend your knees and place your feet in the pockets next to the center pocket of your Core Band. Stretch your feet apart to pull the pocket taut. Place your hands in the end sleeves. Extend your legs toward the ceiling to form a small V.

Movement sequence

1 Round your back and roll onto your shoulder blades, keeping your arms straight. Roll over with your legs straight until they are parallel to the floor over your head. Keep your head up and in line with your spine so it does not initiate the movement or touch the mat.

2 Roll up to your starting position.

Repetitions Repeat 5 times.

Breathing pattern Inhale as you roll back. Exhale as you roll up.

Goal Try to maintain your body design and keep your arms straight as you roll back and up so that the distance from your shoulders to your legs remains equal in all positions. This will ensure that you are doing a core movement and not swinging your legs.

Modifications Placing your feet on the band instead of in the sleeves will make the exercise easier.

Take the core challenge Place your feet in the center pocket and your hands in the sleeves next to them. The closer the hand placement, the more difficult the movement will be.

roll-over

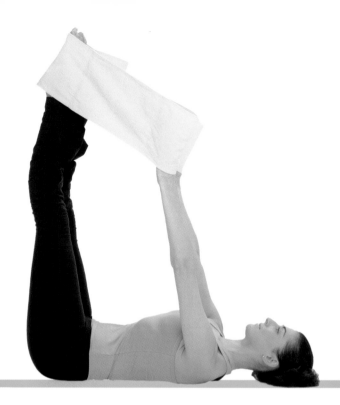

Benefits This exercise works your deepest layer of abdominal muscles and massages your spine. The aim is to place each vertebra on the mat, one at a time, with full spinal control and articulation.

Starting alignment Lie on your mat and place your feet in the center pocket of the Core Band. Slide your hands into the end sleeves with your palms facing inward.

Movement sequence

1   Extend your legs to the ceiling, straightening your arms. Contract your abdominal muscles and roll your tailbone off the mat. Keep pulling your lower abdominal muscles inward and bring your navel to your spine.

2   Keeping your arms straight, continue to roll over, peeling your spine from the floor one vertebra at a time, rolling with control until your legs are overhead and parallel to the floor. Take several deep breaths as you roll.

3   Begin to roll down, placing each vertebra on the mat. Use the band for resistance, keeping your arms straight. Breathe deeply and press the full length of your spine to the mat. Bring your tailbone down and straighten your legs toward the ceiling.

Repetitions Repeat the exercise 5 times.

Breathing pattern Inhale as you extend your legs to the ceiling.

Exhale as you contract your abdominal muscles. Continue breathing deeply as you roll over and down.

Goal Your movement goal is to perform this exercise with complete control. Do not throw your legs

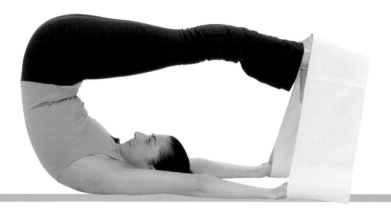

overhead; rather, peel your spine off the floor using deep core contractions, and use the strength of your entire core to roll down one vertebra at a time. Keep your arms straight in order to stabilize your torso. Do not bend your elbows toward your chest. Your feet should remain parallel with the floor and not drop over your head. The roll comes from your core muscles, not from momentum in swinging. Core control and fluid motion are the best ways to stretch your spine.

Modifications If you cannot lift your legs overhead with core control, stretch your toes toward your head and pull into the band for a great stretch. Contract your abdominal muscles and hollow your abdomen, lifting your tailbone off the floor. Press your tailbone down to the floor and repeat, lifting higher each time.

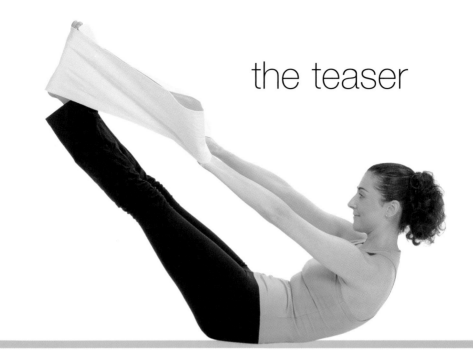

the teaser

Benefits The most beneficial and challenging core work involves the whole body in performing the movement. Movement that is initiated in the core, then radiates into the head and neck, arms and legs is totally connected kinetically.

Starting alignment Lie on your mat and place your feet in the center pocket of the Core Band. Slide your hands into the end sleeves with your palms facing inward.

Movement sequence

1 Extend your legs to the ceiling, straightening your arms. Curl your upper body off the mat, lowering your legs. Keep your arms straight, your shoulders down, and your abdominals contracted.

2 Open your arms out at the sides of your body. Curl your torso toward your legs while lifting your legs higher, stretching upward to a V position.

3 Take a deep breath and begin to roll your torso down away from your legs, keeping your legs lifted. Press your lower back to the floor with a strong abdominal contraction.

4 Curl up to the V position once again, opening your arms out at the sides of your body. Repeat the lower back imprint a few times. Roll your torso down and lower your legs to complete the exercise.

Repetitions Repeat the exercise 5 times.

Breathing pattern Inhale as you extend your legs to the ceiling.

Exhale as you curl your upper body off the mat. Inhale as you open your arms, and exhale as you curl your torso toward your legs.

Breathe deeply as you roll down to your mat.

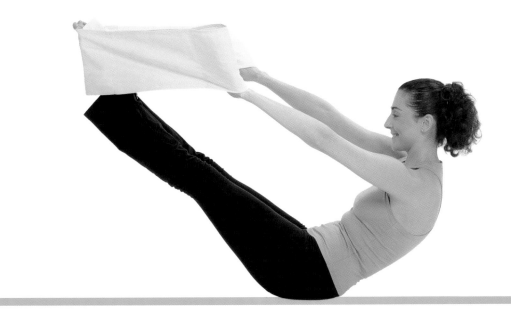

Goal Keep pulling your navel to your spine and press your tailbone to your mat. Do not pop up, but roll slowly and sequentially. As you roll up, keep your lower back pressed to the floor. Do not balance on your tailbone. Lift your chest and lengthen your spine upward for a more advanced stretch.

Modifications Lift your torso only as far as you can without feeling tension in your neck and shoulders. Maintain your core alignment and modify your range of motion to work your core muscles to their maximum potential.

Take the core challenge Perform the Roll-over (pages 88–89) with the Teaser for a dynamic combination of movements.

Challenge your core strength by lowering and lifting your legs from the Teaser position. Keep you upper body still and lower and lift 5 times.

the swan

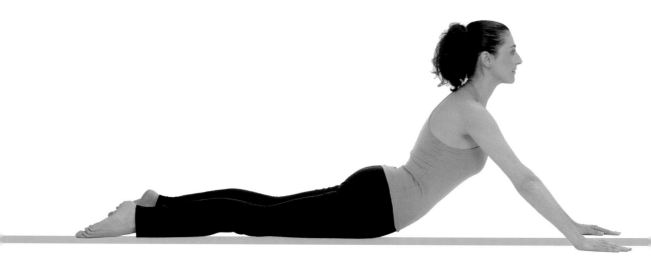

Benefits This extension exercise strengthens your back muscles and improves spinal flexibility.

Starting alignment Lie on your stomach with your forehead on your mat and your arms stretched straight in front of you. Bring your legs hip-distance apart.

Movement sequence

1 Lift your head, neck, and shoulders and slide your arms toward your torso.

2 Pull your shoulder blades down, lengthen your neck, and lift your chest up from the floor.

3 Slowly lower your torso to the floor, stretching from your hips to your rib cage. Place your shoulders and head down.

Repetitions Repeat the exercise 5 times.

Breathing pattern Take a full breath to lift your torso upward.

Hold the stretch for a full breath.

Lower your torso on a third full breath.

Goal Engage your middle back muscles to perform the lift. Keep your abdominals pulled inward for support. Do not arch your neck or the middle of your spine but keep your entire spine lengthened.

Modification Keep your movement controlled from your core muscles. This will prevent you from pushing off the floor with your arms, which can put pressure on your lower back.

swimming

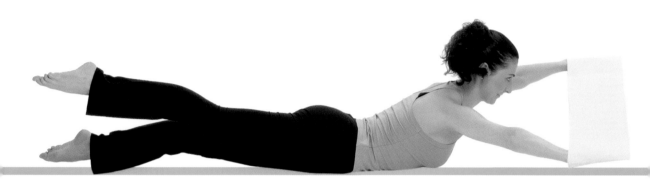

Benefits While the movement in this exercise is in your arms and legs, the main focus is on your core muscles. Maintaining stability in your shoulders and pelvis controls the movements through your whole body.

Starting alignment Lie face down on your mat. Place your hands in the Core Band, using sleeves slightly wider apart than your shoulders. Bring your legs hip-distance apart in a slight turn-out position.

Movement sequence

1   Lift your arms up to eye level and lift your legs up as well.

2   Perform a small flutter motion with your opposite arm and leg. Emphasize the upward motion especially with your back and arm muscles.

Repetitions Perform 30 little kicks.

Breathing pattern Inhale for 5 counts and exhale for 5 counts.

Goal Keep your arms and legs lifted and emphasize the upward motion of the exercise. Do not arch your neck or hunch your shoulders. Keep your shoulder blades pulled away from your ears and keep your band pulled taut.

Modification Increase your repetitions to 50 as you progress. Lessen the number of repetitions if you lose your core control.

kneeling side stretch

Benefits This exercise stretches your oblique muscles and trims your waistline. Your core positioning increases the muscle work and adds joint stability to the movement.

Starting alignment Kneel on your mat with your legs hip-distance apart. Place your hands into the sleeves of the Core Band. Stretch to the side, placing one hand on the floor. Stretch your other hand over your head, pulling the band upward in a vertical line from floor to ceiling. Extend your opposite leg out, placing the side of your foot on the floor. Align your shoulders and your hips, and keep them stable throughout the exercise.

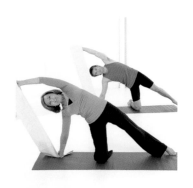

Movement sequence

1   Pull your band upward, reaching toward the ceiling.

2   Release the pull and stretch your band toward the floor, keeping your arm over your head.

3   Pull the band up to the ceiling.

Repetitions Repeat the movement 5 times.

Breathing pattern Inhale as you pull your band upward.

Exhale as you release the pull.

Inhale as you stretch your band toward you.

Exhale as you pull the band up to the ceiling.

Goal Improved torso flexibility, upper body strength, and a toned waistline are the goals of the exercise.

Modifications Sit on the floor with your knees bent to one side of your body. Tuck your feet close to your hips. Extend your top leg out on the floor. Stretch your torso to the opposite side and perform the exercise in this modified position.

Take the core challenge: Lift and lower your outstretched leg, with one full breath, while releasing the pull of the band.

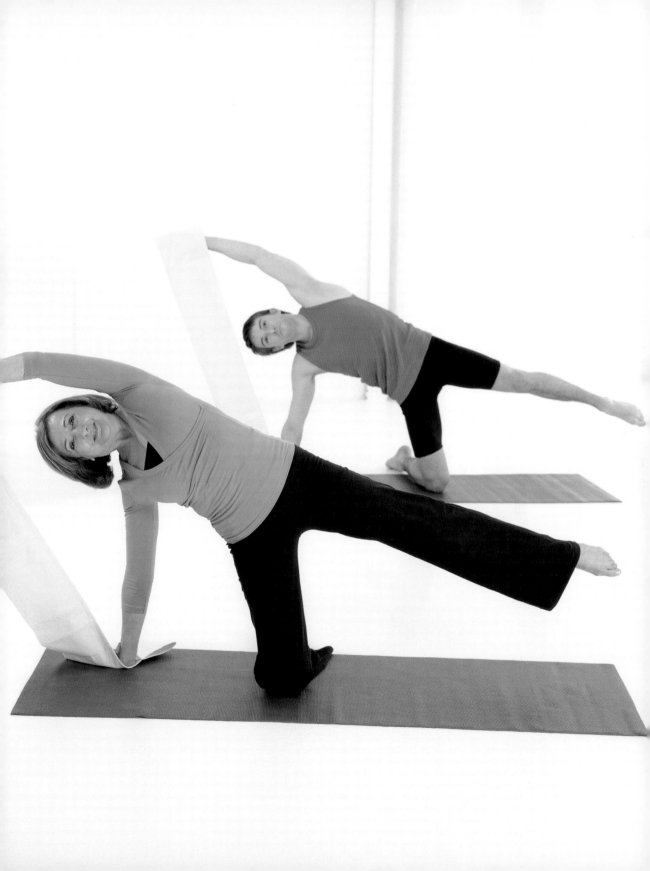

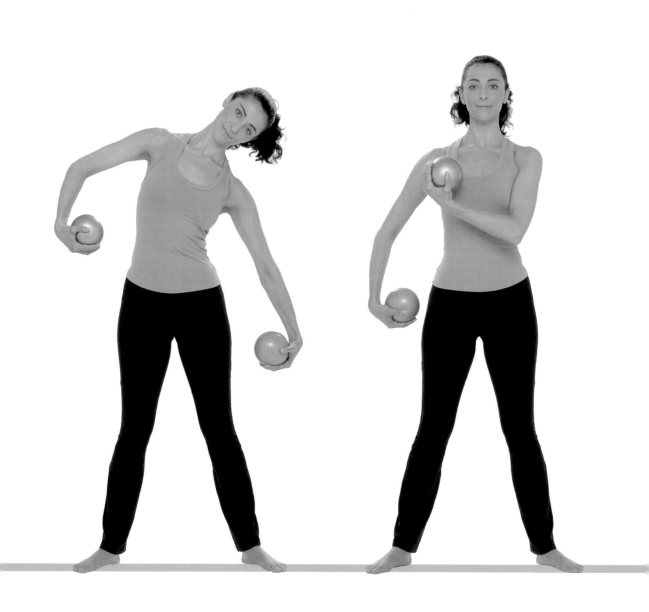

standing side bends with crossed biceps curls

Benefits This exercise trims your waistline and transfers your core work into your arms to strengthen your whole-body connections.

Starting alignment Stand with your feet slightly wider than hip-distance apart. Hold your weights in your hands.

Movement sequence: Standing Side Bends

1   Stretch to one side, bending your opposite arm and lifting your weight up the side of your body.

2   Lower your weight, straightening your torso.

3   Repeat the movement to the other side.

4   Repeat this pattern 2 times.

Movement sequence: Crossed Biceps Curls

1   Bend your elbow and lift your weight across your body to your opposite shoulder.

2   Lower your arm to the side of your body with your palm facing inward.

3   Repeat the movement with your other arm.

4   Do 10 repetitions, alternating arms.

Repetitions Do 3 sets of the entire pattern.

Breathing pattern Inhale and exhale as you bend to your side.

Inhale and exhale as you straighten.

Exhale as you lift your weight.

Inhale as you lower your weight to the side of your body.

Goal Be aware of centering your body from your torso into your arms and legs and how your correct hip and shoulder alignment affects your stance and movement.

Stretch directly to the side. Do not allow your shoulders to twist. Pull the weight up the side of your body, keeping it in contact with your side.

When performing the biceps curl, keep your elbow close to your waistline and reach as far across your chest as you can.

Modifications Reduce the amount of weight and number of repetitions if you cannot complete 1 full set.

Take the core challenge Add more weight when you can easily perform 3 sets of the exercise.

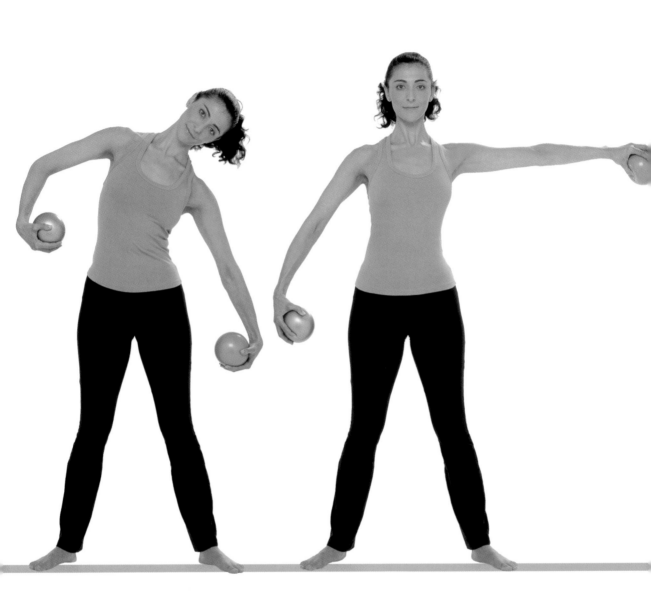

standing side bends with straight arm lifts

Benefits Correct joint alignment produces optimal motion. Your shoulder girdle must be in its neutral position—not elevated, depressed, or forward. Keeping this alignment during this sequence creates muscle balance. It does not over-develop one group at the expense of another.

Starting alignment Stand with your feet slightly wider than hip-distance apart. Hold your weights in your hands.

Movement sequence: Standing Side Bends

1 Stretch to one side, bending your opposite arm and lifting your weight up the side of your body.
2 Lower your weight, straightening your torso.
3 Repeat the movement to the other side.
4 Repeat this pattern 2 times.

Movement sequence: Straight Arm Lifts

1 Lift one arm up at the side of your body.
2 Lower your arm to the side of your body with your palm facing inward.
3 Repeat the movement with your other arm.
4 Lift both arms up at the sides of your body.
5 Lower both arms.
6 Do 5 sets of Straight Arm Lifts.

Repetitions Do 3 sets of the entire pattern.

Breathing pattern Inhale and exhale as you bend to your side.
Inhale and exhale as you straighten.
Exhale as you lift your weight.
Inhale as you lower your weight to the side of your body.

Goal Stretch directly to the side. Do not allow your shoulders to twist. Pull the weight up the side of your body, keeping it in contact with your side. When performing the Straight Arm Lifts, start with your less dominant arm to create a balance in your motion.

Modifications Reduce the amount of weight and number of repetitions if you cannot complete 1 full set.

Take the core challenge Add more weight when you can easily perform 3 sets of the exercise.

deltoid fly

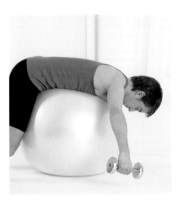

Benefits The Deltoid Fly strengthens the back of your shoulders and upper back muscles. It improves your posture and trains your core muscles to aid your arm muscles. Lying over a stability ball reduces the risk of arching your back.

Starting alignment Round your torso over your stability ball, belly first, with your feet on the floor, hip-distance apart, and your knees bent. Hold your hand weights in your hands and hug the sides of the ball. Maintain your core alignment and do not allow your shoulders or hips to sink into the ball. Stabilize your core and keep all your muscles active to stabilize the ball.

Movement sequence

1 Lift your arms up at the sides of your body to shoulder level.
2 Stretch your arms wide and lower them around the ball.

Repetitions Repeat 10 times.

Breathing pattern Exhale as you lift your arms.
Inhale as you lower your arms.

Goal Make sure not to lock your arms. Bend your elbows slightly as you lift. Bring your shoulder blades together as you lift and fully broaden your back as you lower your arms. Keep your head down and in line with your spine.

Modifications If your shoulders are weak, minimize your range of motion and lessen your weights. The point is to build a strength system from within, not to tear down the connections.

Take the core challenge Complete 3 sets of movements.

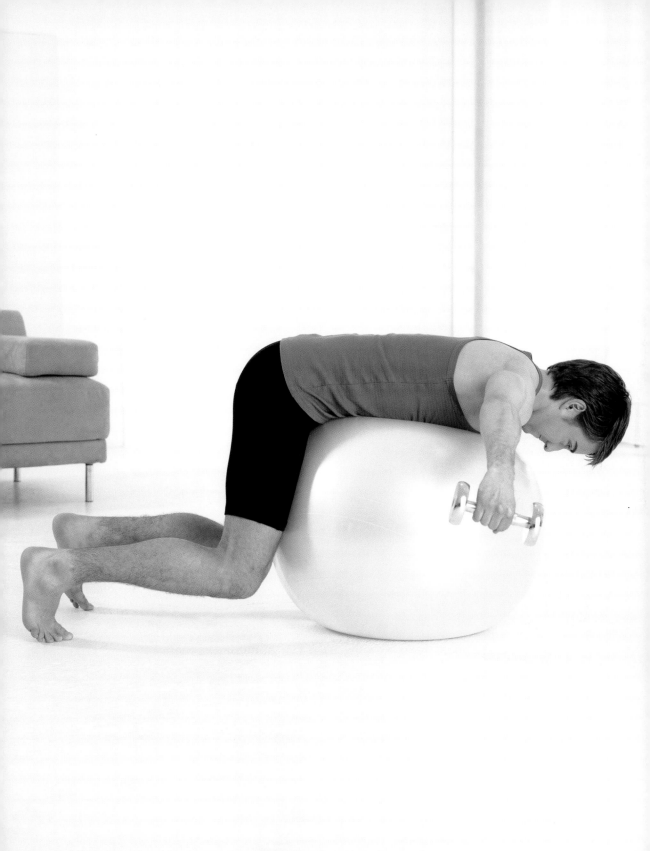

abdominal curls with arm extensions

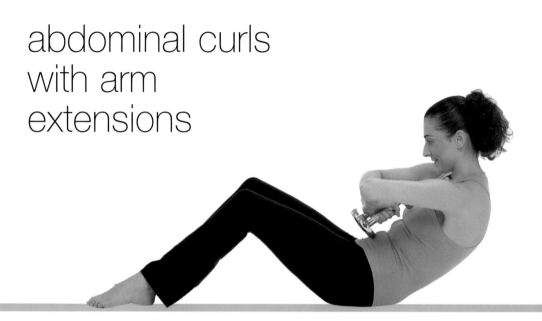

Benefits Adding weights and arm extensions to your abdominal curl checks if you are cheating and losing your core alignment in the movement. Keep your abdominals pulled inward and your abdomen concave throughout the exercise.

Starting alignment Sit on your mat with your knees bent and feet flat. Bring your feet hip-distance apart and hold your weights in your hands with your palms down. Bend your arms and place the weights on your rib cage with your elbows open to the sides of your body.

Movement sequence

1 Contract your abdominals and begin to curl down to the floor one vertebra at a time. As you roll, stretch your arms out in front of you at chest level. Roll down to your shoulder blades.

2 Open your arms out at the sides of your body.

3 Close your arms in front of your chest.

4 Curl up from your mat, bending your arms and pulling the weights to your rib cage.

Repetitions Repeat the exercise 5 times.

Breathing pattern Take a full breath to curl down to your mat.

Inhale as you open your arms.

Exhale to bring them together.

Take a full breath to curl up to sitting.

Goal Your goal is precision in motion. Place each vertebra to your mat with control, and extend your arms slowly away from your body. As you curl up, visualize pulling your abdominals away from your weights as they come toward your torso.

Modifications Curl down only as far as you can without losing the curl of your spine and abdominal contraction. If your abdominals push out,

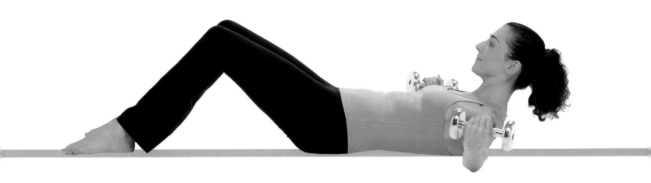

you have lost your pelvic alignment, which can lead to back strain.

Do not extend your arms, keeping the weights on your rib cage as you curl down and up.

Take the core challenge Add 4 arm extensions in the curled-down position before curling up. Curl up 1 inch farther from your mat. Hold this position and perform the exercise. Curl down and repeat the arm extensions. Slowly curl up 2 inches farther from your mat and repeat the exercise. Keep repeating the pattern, curling up 1 inch farther each time. Maintain your core alignment and deep abdominal contraction to work with specificity and control

oblique curls with arm extensions

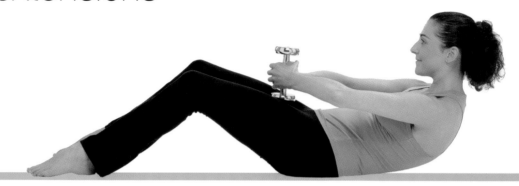

Benefits The torso rotation in this exercise increases spinal flexibility and works the oblique muscles, which run along your sides.

Starting alignment Sit on your mat with your knees bent and feet flat. Bring your feet hip-distance apart and hold one weight in your hands with your palms facing each other. Bend your arms and place the weight on your rib cage with your elbows open to the sides of your body.

Movement sequence

1 Contract your abdominals and begin to curl down to the floor one vertebra at a time. As you roll, stretch your arms out in front of you at chest level. Roll down to your shoulder blades.

2 Rotate your upper torso to one side of your body, stretching your arms away from your torso, keeping your abdominals contracted and your arms straight.

3 Bend your arms and pull your weight to your chest.

4 Extend your arms out at the side of your body.

5 Bring your arms into the center position.

6 Curl up from your mat, bending your arms and pulling the weights to your rib cage.

7 Repeat the exercise, curling to the other side.

Repetitions Repeat the exercise 6 times.

Breathing pattern Take a full breath to curl down to your mat.

Inhale as you curl to the side.

Exhale and bring your arms to your chest.

Inhale to straighten your arms.

Exhale as you curl your torso center.

Take a full breath to curl up to sitting.

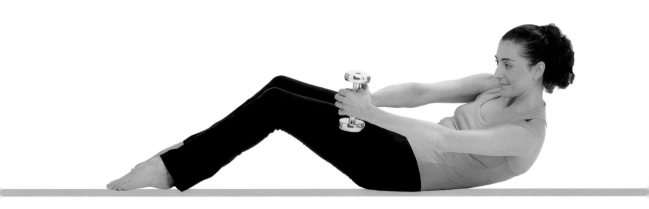

Goal Do not change your pelvic alignment as you curl to the side. Keep both hips anchored as you twist. Make sure to maintain your shoulder alignment as you rotate. The movement comes from your core. Feel the twist in your waistline, not from your shoulders. Your top shoulder should not lift from your ear and your breastbone should remain lifted as you rotate. Concentrate on using your breath to increase the intensity of the arm extensions.

Modifications You may want to try this exercise without the weights. Cross your arms across your chest, placing your opposite hands on your shoulders. Omit the arm extensions and concentrate on feeling the rotation of your core muscles.

Take the core challenge Add 4 arm extensions in the curled-down position before curling up. Add more repetitions, then more weight to progress.

cobra pose
Bhujangasana

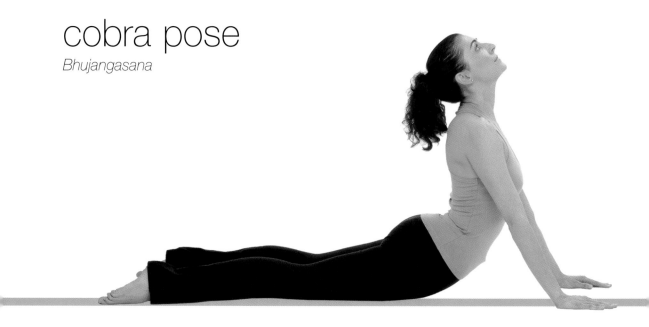

Benefits The Cobra Pose opens your chest and stretches your back muscles and is the remedy for long hours spent at the computer or in your car. This exercise strengthens the long muscles in your back and between your shoulder blades.

Starting alignment Lie on your stomach with your forehead on your mat. Bring your legs together and point your feet. Place your hands palms-down under your shoulders. Keep your elbows bent, close to the sides of your body.

Movement sequence

1 Pull your shoulder blades down, away from your ears, and lift your head and chest from your mat.

2 Lift your chest and back upward, extending from your pelvis to the top of your head.

3 Stretch your torso toward the floor, imprinting the

front of your body, and keeping your spine elongated as you lower.

Repetitions Perform the Cobra Pose twice.

Breathing pattern Inhale and exhale as you stretch upward.

Stay in the pose for 3 full breaths.

Lower your torso with an inhalation and long exhalation.

Goal Your movement must come from your torso, not from pressing with your arms. Lift with your back muscles and only use your arms to aid your stretch. Never arch your neck or tilt your head back. Your stretch is a movement forward and upward.

Modification For a more gentle stretch, place your forearms on the floor under your shoulders and keep your navel on your mat to increase the stretch into your upper back.

bow pose

Dhanurasana

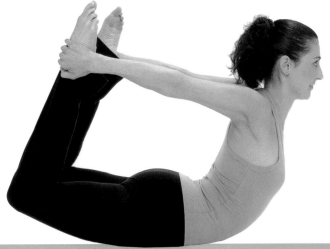

Benefits Following the Cobra (see opposite), the Bow Pose adds an extra stretch into the front of your thighs while at the same time opening your chest. The stretch of the front of your body also aids digestion.

Starting alignment Lie on your mat on your stomach. Bring your feet apart slightly, keeping your legs parallel. Place your hands on the floor at the sides of your body with your palms up.

Movement sequence

1   Bend one leg and bring your foot toward your torso. Lift your matching arm and hold your foot.

2   Repeat this movement with your other foot and arm.

3   Lift your torso and knees upward, stretching equally through your core. Press your pelvis into your mat as you increase the upward movement.

4   Lower your knees, release your feet, and relax your chest onto the mat.

Repetitions Do the Bow Pose 3 times.

Breathing pattern Take a full breath to hold your feet.

Inhale and exhale to stretch upward.

Stay in the pose for 3 full breaths.

Release the pose with long, full breath.

Goal The goal is to lengthen your torso and stretch from your pelvis to the top of your head while lifting your thighs high off the mat. Raise your arms toward the ceiling without pulling your legs up. The muscle work needs to be initiated from your core.

Modification Place a rolled blanket under your hips. Reach back, bend one leg, and hold one foot in your hand. Release and repeat with your other leg. Repeat, holding both legs and keeping your knees on the floor.

stability ball pelvic curls

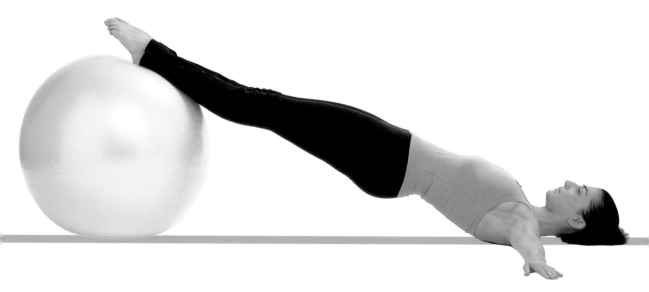

Benefits Your spinal articulation is tested in this exercise. The stability ball will roll if you are not performing this movement from your core.

Starting alignment Lie on the floor, bend your knees, and place your feet on top of the ball. Bring your feet hip-distance apart and stretch your arms out at the sides of your body at shoulder level with your palms down.

Movement sequence

1   Roll your spine up off the floor one vertebra at a time from your tailbone to your shoulder blades while straightening your legs and rolling the ball away from your torso.

2   Curl down, imprinting your back to the floor while bending your knees and pulling the ball toward your torso.

Repetitions Repeat the exercise 5 times.

Breathing pattern Take 2 full breaths to curl up. Hold your lifted position for 1 breath. Inhale and exhale twice as you roll down.

Goal Control from your core is the goal. Articulate your spine as you feel the fluidity of the roll of the ball. Make sure to roll both hips evenly and not arch your back. Maintain your cross-point alignment through your torso as you roll up and down.

Modifications Place your feet on the floor and roll without the ball. You may want to increase your stability by placing the ball a few inches away from the wall. When you are in the extended position, the ball will not roll away from your torso.

Take the core challenge To really deepen your core muscle work, keep your knees bent as you roll up and down. Do not change your leg position or allow the ball to move at all during the exercise.

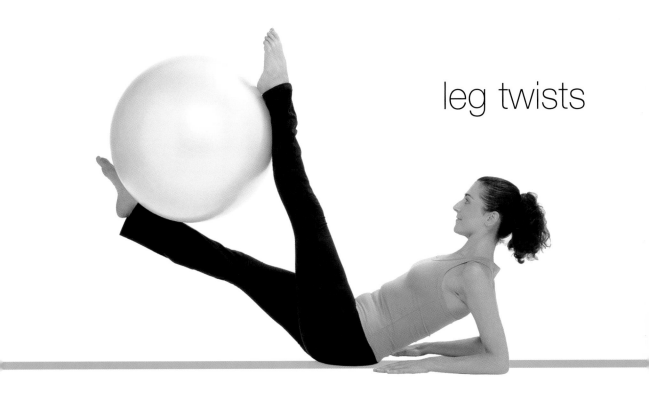

leg twists

Benefits This movement opens your hips and works your abdominals and inner and outer thighs.

Starting alignment Sit on the floor, resting on your elbows. Keep your legs straight and hold the ball between your ankles. Contract your abdominal muscles and press your lower back into the floor.

Movement sequence

1 Lift the ball off the floor and raise your legs on a diagonal to the ceiling.

2 Twist from your hips, bringing one leg toward your chest while the other leg circles away from your torso.

3 Reverse and circle the other way.

Repetitions Repeat the exercise 10 times.

Breathing pattern Take a full breath to complete each circle.

Goal Do not allow your pelvis to tilt. Your goal is to lower your legs slightly with each circle, maintaining the control from your abdominals and pelvis.

Modifications Keep your legs high to maintain your pelvic alignment and reduce the number of repetitions. Squeeze your inner thigh muscles to hold on to the stability ball.

straight leg lifts
in plank position

Benefits You will test your core pelvic alignment in this movement. Your body awareness, focus, and concentration are called upon to steady the ball from your inner structure.

Starting alignment Lie on the floor, and place your feet on top of the ball with your legs straight. Stretch your arms out at the sides of your body at shoulder level with your palms down.

Movement sequence

1 Roll your spine up off the floor one vertebra at a time from your tailbone to your shoulder blades. Keep your legs straight and the ball stable.

2 Lift one leg to the ceiling, keeping your leg straight and hips level. Lower your leg to touch the ball without rolling. Perform the movement with the same leg 5 times.

3 Repeat the exercise with the other leg.

4 Curl down, imprinting your back to the floor while keeping your legs straight and the ball stable.

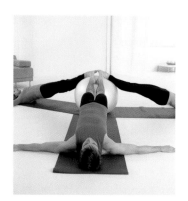

Repetitions Repeat the exercise 2 times.

Breathing pattern Take 2 full breaths to curl up.

Exhale as you lift your leg.

Inhale as you lower your leg.

Inhale and exhale twice as you roll down.

Goal Pelvic stability is your movement goal. Take care to keep your hips stable. Do not let them roll as you lift and lower.

Modifications You may want to place the ball against the wall when you first start this movement. Progress when you feel your hips do not move as you lift your legs.

Take the core challenge Alternate lifting one leg then the other without transferring your body weight from side to side as you lift and lower.

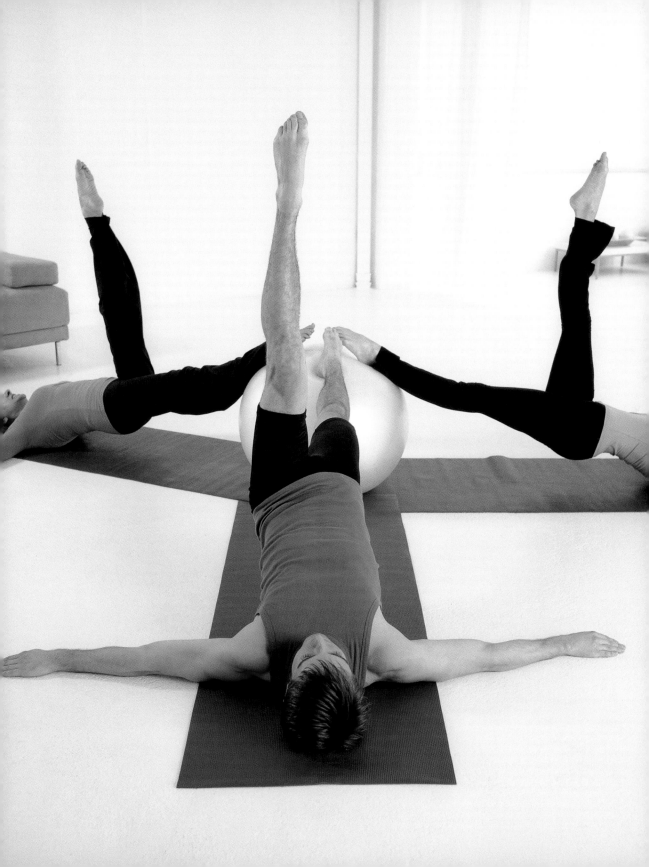

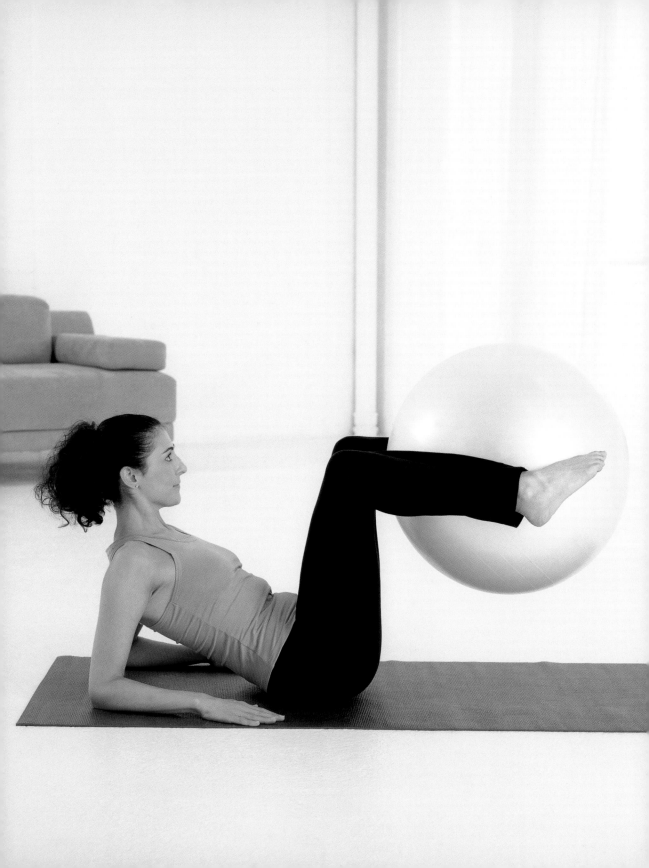

leg extensions

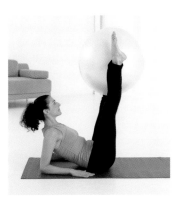

Benefits This exercise builds your abdominal control and helps you to focus on how your core muscles are affected by all your movements.

Starting alignment Sit on the floor, resting on your elbows. Hold the ball between your ankles. Contract your abdominal muscles and press your lower back into the floor.

Movement sequence

1 Lift the ball off the floor and bend your knees toward your chest.

2 Extend your legs toward the ceiling.

3 Bend your knees toward your chest.

4 Extend your legs out as close to the floor as you can while maintaining your core alignment.

Repetitions Repeat the exercise 10 times.

Breathing pattern Inhale as you bend your knees.

Exhale as you extend your legs up.

Inhale as you bend your knees.

Exhale as you extend your legs out.

Goal Do not allow your pelvis to tilt as you extend your legs out.

This will take a great deal of abdominal control. Keep your chest lifted.

Do not sink into your elbows or shoulders.

Modifications As you extend your legs, keep them higher to maintain your pelvic alignment. Reduce the number of repetitions and use your core muscles to support the leg work.

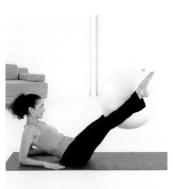

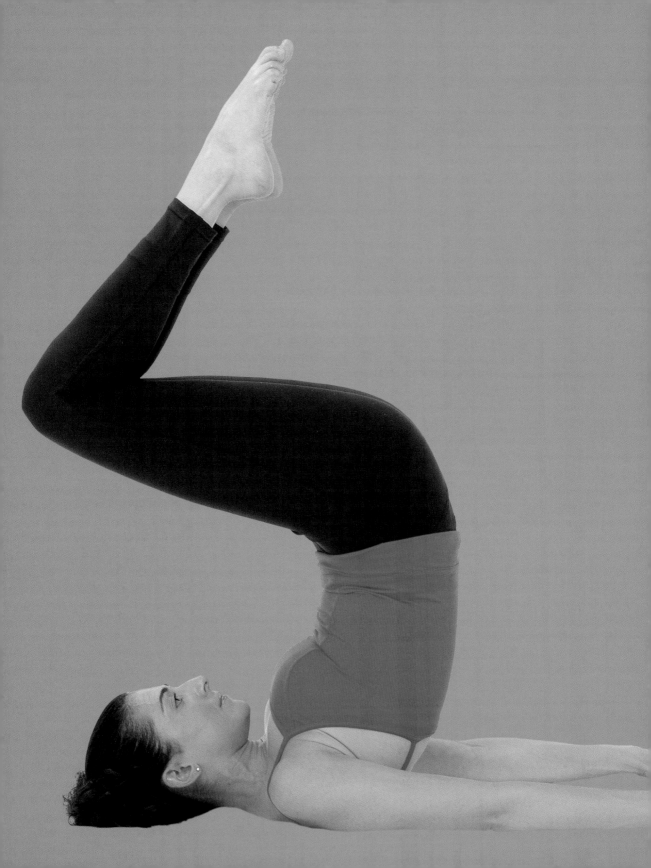

program 3

The Total Core Challenge

This is an exciting program for those advancing in their core fitness training. Through higher-energy exercises, dynamic movement sequences, and advanced breath work, you will progress to meet ambitious fitness goals. This is a challenging, rewarding, and effective program for precision training for life.

stability ball imprint

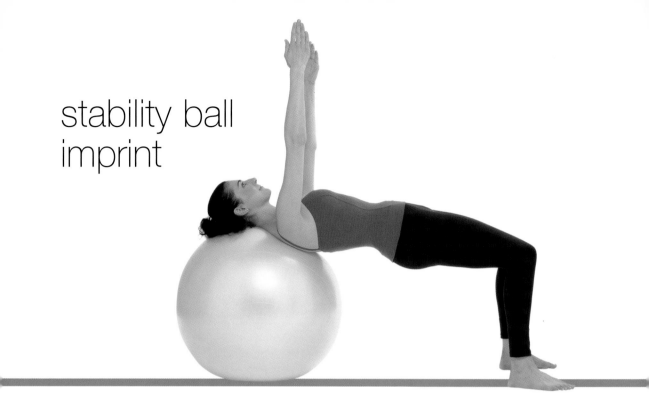

Benefits Imprinting your spine while rolling on the ball massages your spine and works your abdominal muscles. Place each vertebra on the ball "like the spokes of a wheel" for full articulation.

Starting alignment Sit on top of the ball with your feet hip-distance apart. Place your hands on the ball at the sides of your torso.

Movement sequence

1 Lift your arms to shoulder level in front of your chest. Contract your abdominals and begin to walk your feet away from the ball as you press your spine into the ball one vertebra at a time.

2 Continue to walk your feet out until your head, neck, and shoulders are on the ball.

3 Keeping your back straight and your hips up, breathe into the stretch.

4 Curl your spine off the ball, walking your feet in to the ball as you round up to sitting.

Repetitions Repeat 3 times.

Breathing pattern Take 3 breaths to walk out. Inhale and exhale twice in the stretch. Take 3 breaths to roll up to sitting.

Goal Do not allow your hips to lower as you walk out or back. Your movement goal is to lengthen your spine as you stretch. Your pelvis does not lower as it leaves the ball for core alignment.

Modifications Walk out only as far as you can with your hips up.

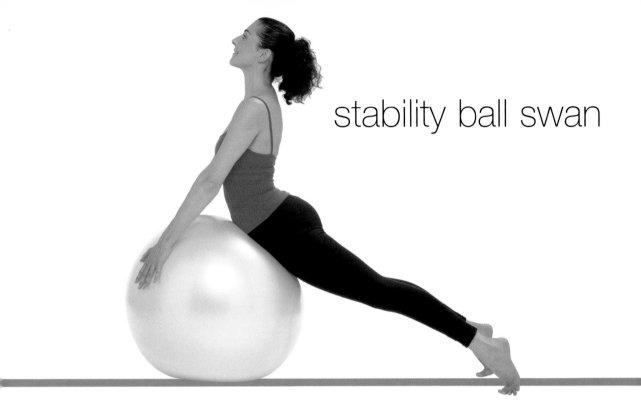

stability ball swan

Benefits Remember how flexible you were as a child? Rolling, twisting, and jumping in all directions was never a problem. As we age, our spines become more rigid. Extension exercises such as this one alleviate stiff backs and create healthier back alignment.

Starting alignment Lie over your ball on your stomach, pressing your pelvis on top. Straighten your legs behind you and bring them hip-distance apart. Curl your toes under for more stability. Place your hands on the ball directly under your shoulders.

Movement sequence

1   Press your shoulder blades down away from your ears and lift your torso upward off the ball. Straighten your arms and lift your navel away from the ball.

2   Gently lower your pelvis, waist, and chest to the ball. Relax your shoulders, neck, and head as you release.

Repetitions Repeat the movement 5 times.

Breathing pattern Lift upward on a full breath. Lower to the ball on a full breath.

Goal Lengthening your spine in extension is your movement goal—not arching your back. Make sure to keep your head in line with your spine so your gaze is straight ahead and your movement is sequential.

Modifications Kneel on the floor or work with your legs wider apart for a firmer base.

spine stretch and twist

Benefits This feel-good exercise makes your back more supple. This is a great way to unwind after a long drive or hours at the computer.

Starting alignment Sit on the floor in front of your stability ball with your knees bent and your feet flat on the floor. Bring your knees and feet hip-distance apart. Hold the sides of the ball with your hands.

Movement sequence: Spine Stretch

1   Lift your arms to shoulder level in front of your chest. Stretch your head, neck, and shoulders to the ball. Slowly begin to wrap your torso over the ball, straightening your legs. Stretch back as far as you can until your legs are fully extended. Hold your arms straight up, pointing to the ceiling.

2   Roll down, bending your knees until you are sitting on the floor.

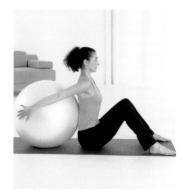

Movement sequence: Twist

After repeating the spine stretch 3 times, add the twist:

1   Roll back on your ball and extend your legs fully. Place one hand on the floor with your palm down.

2   Turn and face your hand, bringing your other arm on top of it.

3   Roll across your shoulder blades, lifting your top arm to the ceiling.

4   Release your other arm from the floor and lift it toward the ceiling.

5   Repeat the twist to the other side.

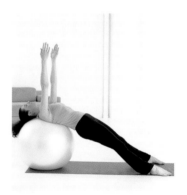

Repetitions Perform 3 Spine Stretches.

Perform 4 Twists, alternating sides.

Breathing pattern Take 3 breaths to roll up.

Take 3 breaths to roll down.

Inhale to lower your arm to the floor.

Exhale to stretch your other arm over.

Inhale to lift your top arm.

Exhale to bring your other arm up.

Goal A balanced, uniform stretch on both sides of your body is your movement goal. If one side is not as stable, work this side first.

Modifications You may need to hold the ball as you start to roll up.

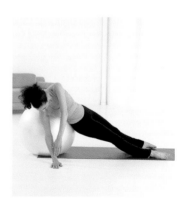

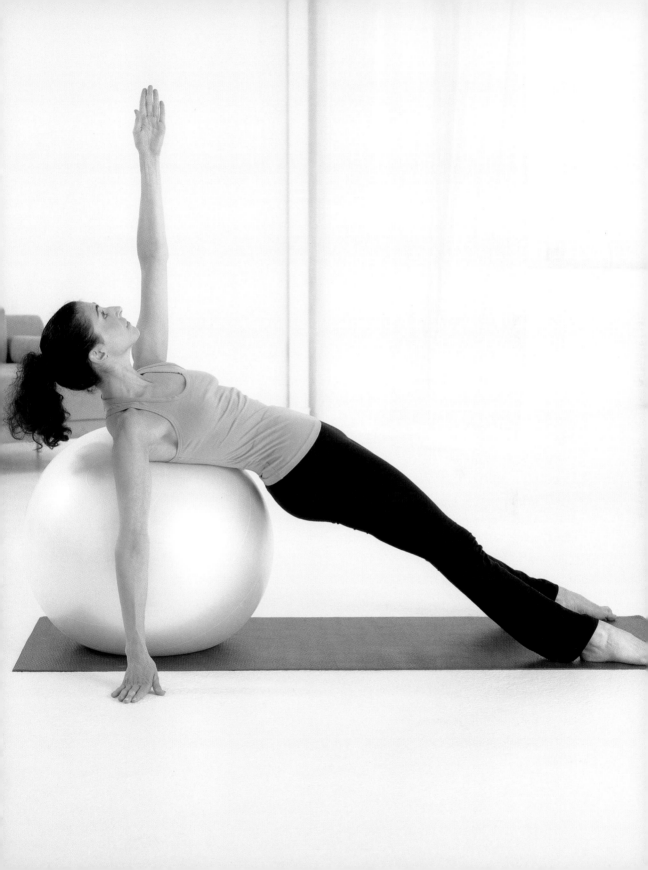

push-ups and leg beats

Benefits Your core muscles remain engaged, yet you work your arms with these push-ups and your legs with small beats.

Starting alignment Lie on top of your stability ball, stomach first, with your legs together and straight. Point your toes. Place your hands on the floor and walk forward until your thighs are resting on top of the ball. Your fingertips should be angled inward. Form a straight line from your shoulders to your wrists.

Movement sequence: Push-ups

1   Keeping your torso still, bend your arms out at the sides of your body, maintaining your plank position.

2   Straighten your arms.

Movement sequence: Leg Beats

1   After performing a push-up, lower your arms toward the floor and lift your legs toward the ceiling. Separate your legs until they are slightly wider than your hips.

2   Close and open your legs with small, quick beats.

3   Bring your legs together and lower them until they are level with the ball.

4   Straighten your arms and walk them back to bring your torso onto the ball.

Repetitions Repeat the Push-up 10 times.

Perform 100 small Leg Beats with your legs.

Breathing pattern Inhale as you bend your arms.

Exhale as you straighten your arms.

Inhale twice and exhale twice as you perform the small beats.

To increase lung capacity, inhale for 5 beats and exhale for 5 beats.

Goal Feel how the engagement of your core muscles lessens the fatigue in your arms and legs as you work at this more intense level.

Take the core challenge Walk your arms out until only your lower leg rests on the ball for your push-ups. Try placing one arm on your back and performing single-arm push-ups.

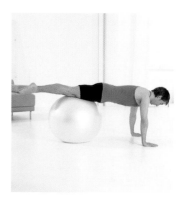

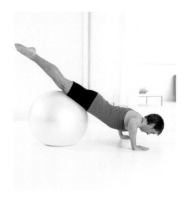

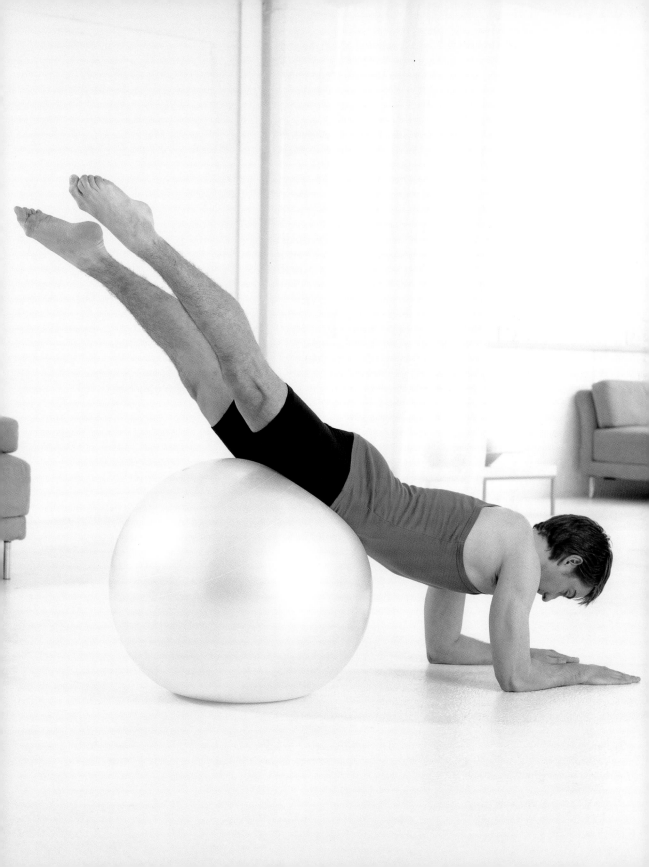

twist with
arm pulls

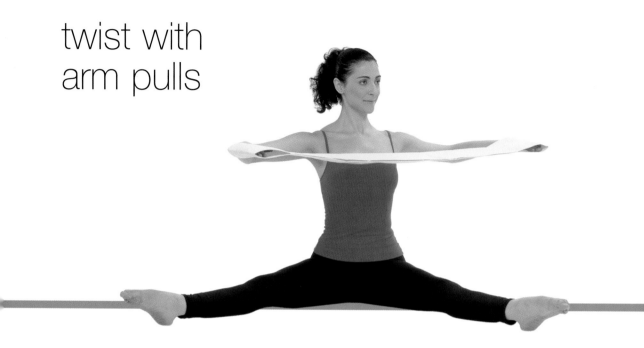

Benefits Rotating your spine and stretching your back muscles corrects misalignments. If one side is tighter than the other, stretch your tight side first.

Starting alignment Sit on your mat with your legs extended out in front of you. Place your hands in the sleeves of the Core Band. Open your legs to a wide V.

Movement sequence

1 Lift your band to chest level.

2 Flex your feet and twist your torso to one side. Keep both hips anchored to your mat, your arms straight, and your band pulled taut.

3 Pull the band to your chest, holding your elbows up at shoulder level.

4 Straighten your arms in front of your chest.

Repetitions Perform 5 repetitions on one side before twisting to center and performing

5 repetitions on the other. Repeat the sequence.

Breathing pattern Take two full breaths to twist your torso.

Inhale as you pull the band to your chest.

Exhale as you extend your arms.

Take two full breaths to twist your torso to the center position.

Goal Elongate your spine and sit up tall out of your hips. Keep both hips pressed to your mat and your abdominal muscles pulled inward and upward. Keep your shoulders down, and allow your head to turn to the side with each twist.

Modifications If your hamstrings are tight, you may want to bend one leg and twist to the straight leg.

Take the core challenge Add single-arm pulls after the double-arm pulls, alternating from the back arm to the front arm.

hip circles

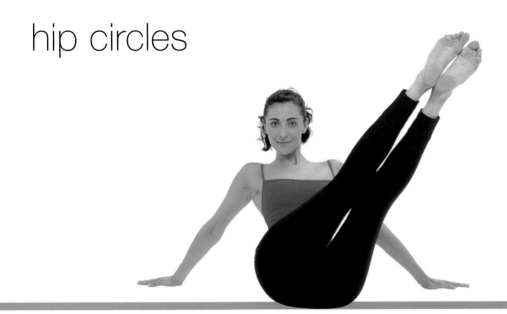

Benefits Abdominal control and core coordination are solidly tested in this exercise. Actively engage all your core muscles and maintain your body design as you circle your legs.

Starting alignment Sit on your mat. Place your arms behind you with your palms down. Bend your knees to your chest. Extend both legs to the ceiling, keeping your toes, ankles, and knees together.

Movement sequence

1   Circle your legs in a clockwise direction, down toward the mat but without touching the mat. Keep your legs straight, with knees and ankles together. Perform 5 circles.

2   Circle your legs to the other side of your torso, this time pulling them up as high as possible. Perform 5 circles.

Repetitions Perform 1 set of circles in this clockwise direction, then another set in a counterclockwise direction.

Breathing pattern Inhale as you circle down. Exhale as you circle upward.

Goal Do not sink into your hands or let your shoulders hunch forward. Your chest should stay lifted and your arms should remain straight as you circle. Maintain your core alignment, keeping your abdominals contracted and your torso stable as you circle your legs.

Modifications You may want to start on your elbows instead of with straight arms. Make your circles very small, and progress only to the point where they remain controlled. Never swing your legs upward, arching your back.

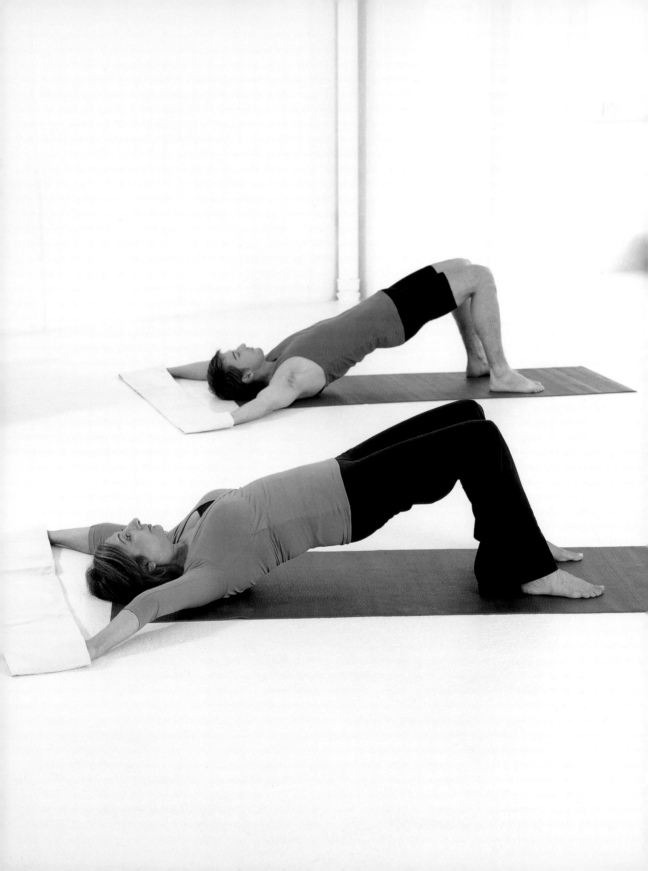

the bridge

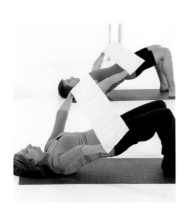

Benefits The Bridge focuses on toning your legs and buttock muscles through the centering of your core.

Starting alignment Lie on your mat with your knees bent and your toes, ankles, and knees together. Place your hands in your Core Band with your arms slightly wider than shoulder-distance apart. Place your arms on the floor over your head.

Movement sequence

1 Roll your spine from your mat, one vertebra at a time, lifting your pelvis up to form a straight line from your shoulders to your hips to your knees.

2 Lift your arms to the ceiling and then reach them to your thighs, keeping them straight all the while.

3 Lift your arms to the ceiling and place them on the floor over your head.

4 Extend one leg and lift it toward the ceiling.

5 Lower your leg to the point at which it is level with your other knee, keeping it straight.

6 Lift your arms to the ceiling and reach them to your thighs.

7 Lift your arms to the ceiling then on the floor over your head.

8 Bend your leg and place your foot on the floor with your legs together.

9 Lift your other leg and repeat the arm stretch.

10 Bend your leg and place your foot on the floor with your toes, ankles, and knees together.

11 Roll your spine down to your mat, one vertebra at a time.

Repetitions Repeat the sequence 3 times.

Breathing pattern Inhale and exhale to roll your spine up.

Inhale as you lift your arms to the ceiling and exhale as you reach to your thighs or to the floor.

Take 2 full breaths to roll your spine down.

Goal Core stability with complete range of motion through your shoulder girdle is your goal. Do not move your hips. Do not kick or swing your leg.

the boomerang

Benefits This dynamic exercise works all parts of your body. Crossing your legs changes your hip alignment while equalizing both sides of your body.

Starting alignment Lie on the floor with your hands at your sides, palms down. Cross one leg on top of the other.

Movement sequence

1 Lift your legs straight toward the ceiling.

2 Bring your legs over your head, stretching back until they are parallel to the floor.

3 Uncross your legs, bringing them to a V position only as wide as your shoulders.

4 Re-cross your legs, placing your other leg on top.

5 Roll your spine down to the floor.

6 Roll your torso up toward your legs as you lower your legs to a diagonal position and lift your arms straight toward your toes.

7 Circle your arms behind your back and clasp your fingers together.

8 Slowly, with complete core control, lower your crossed, straight legs to the floor, reaching your torso toward your legs and your arms back and up toward the ceiling.

9 Unclasp your hands and circle them around toward your toes.

10 Roll your torso up to a sitting position.

Repetitions Perform the Boomerang sequence 5 times.

Breathing pattern Inhale to lift your legs.

Exhale to roll over.

Take a quick breath to uncross and re-cross your legs.

Take 2 breaths to roll up.

Fully inhale and exhale as you circle your arms behind your back.

Take 3 full breaths as you lower your legs and stretch your arms upward.

Inhale and exhale twice as you roll up to a sitting position.

Goal The challenge is controlled strength, flexibility, and precision of movement. Keep your abdominals scooped at all times and do not use momentum to roll over or up.

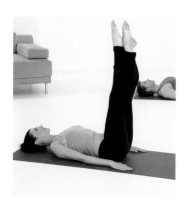

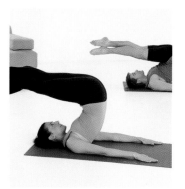

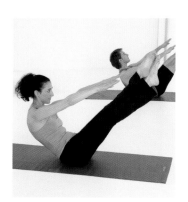

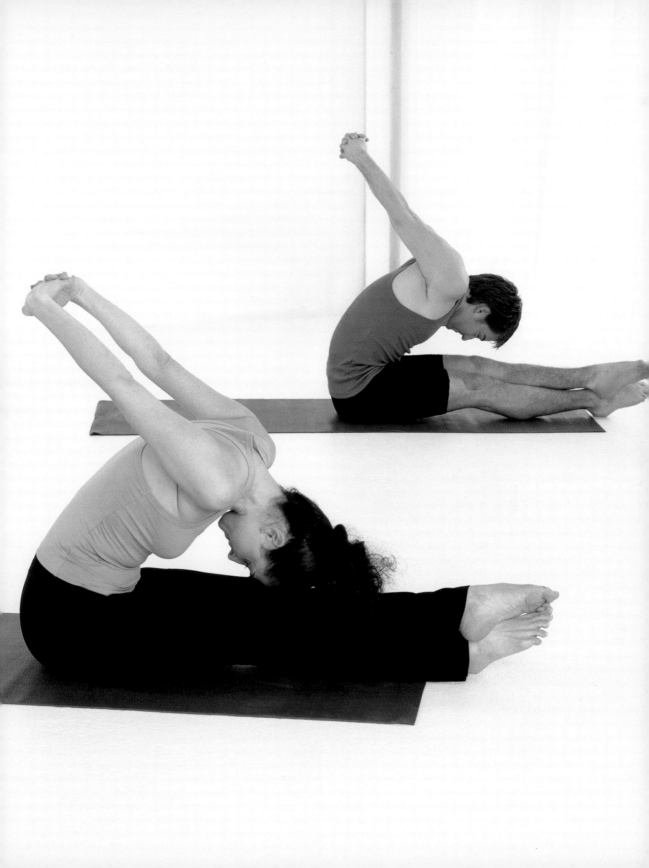

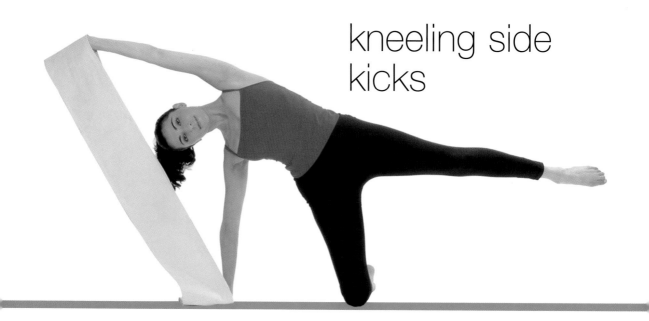

kneeling side kicks

Benefits This exercise challenges your balance, strength, and flexibility. It is an advanced movement, and the Core Band makes it even more challenging.

Starting alignment Kneel on your mat with your legs hip-distance apart. Place your hands into the sleeves of the Core Band. Stretch to the side, placing one hand on the floor. Stretch your other hand over your head, pulling the band upward in a vertical line from floor to ceiling. Extend your opposite leg out, placing the side of your foot on the floor.

Movement sequence

1 Lift your leg so it is level with your hip and parallel to the floor.

2 Sweep your leg in front of your torso without moving your hips or your shoulders. Sweep only

as far as you can without swaying or allowing the band to move.

3 Sweep your leg backward, keeping it hip-distance above your mat at all times.

Repetitions Perform 5 repetitions before repeating with your other leg.

Breathing pattern Inhale as you sweep your leg in front of your torso.
Exhale as you sweep it back.

Goal Your goal is to maintain the equal height of your leg from the front to the side and back. Keep your band pulled taut, and do not allow it to sway as you sweep your leg. Align your shoulders and hips, and keep them stable throughout the exercise. Do not lean into your supporting arm. Keep a straight line from your shoulder to your hand on the floor. Your oblique muscles support your torso. Make sure

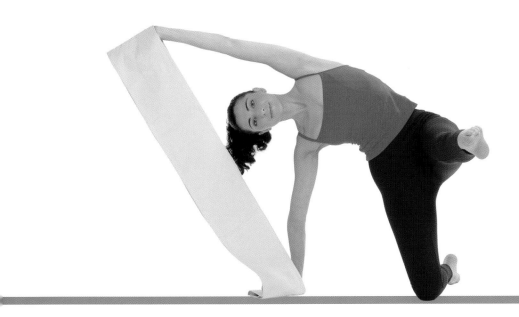

your head stays in line with your spine and you are looking directly ahead, not down to the floor or up to the ceiling. If you are looking at the floor or the ceiling, your neck is out of alignment.

Modifications Minimize your range of motion to keep your movement controlled. Concentrate on your form and body alignment rather than how far you can sweep your leg.

Take the core challenge Perform the exercises in the Side Kick Series (see pages 63–64) in this position for an extra challenge.

the twist

Benefits The Twist works your abdominals and waistline and stretches your spine. It strengthens your upper body and improves your balance.

Starting alignment Place your hands in the pockets of the Core Band. Sit with your knees bent to one side of your body. Cross your top foot over your bottom foot. Place your opposite hand on the floor, keeping your arm straight.

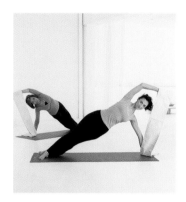

Movement sequence

1　Press your hips upward as you extend and straighten your legs. Lift your top arm over your head.
2　Round your back and contract your abdominals. Twist from your hips, turning your top hip toward your mat. Bring your top arm down and stretch it under your torso, sweeping the band toward the floor.
3　Twist your hips into the center position, bringing your arm up and pulling the band into the vertical position.
4　Open your chest toward the ceiling and stretch your arm back, allowing your gaze to follow your band. Keep pulling the band taut.
5　Twist back to center position. Repeat this movement pattern 3 times.
6　Lower your hips, bending your knees, and sit down on your mat.

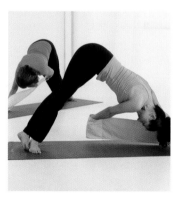

Repetitions Perform the pattern once on each side.

Breathing pattern Inhale as you press your hips upward as you extend and straighten your legs.

Exhale as you twist and sweep the band toward the floor.

Inhale and twist center.

Exhale and open your chest toward the ceiling.

Inhale and twist to center.

Exhale to lower your hips.

Goal The goal is to make sure your twist comes from your hips, not your legs or feet. Allow your head to follow your top arm as you twist and reach.

Modifications Perform the exercise in a kneeling position. Kneel on one knee. Extend the other leg out at the side of your body with your foot on the floor.

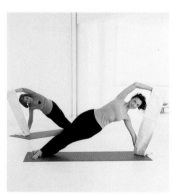

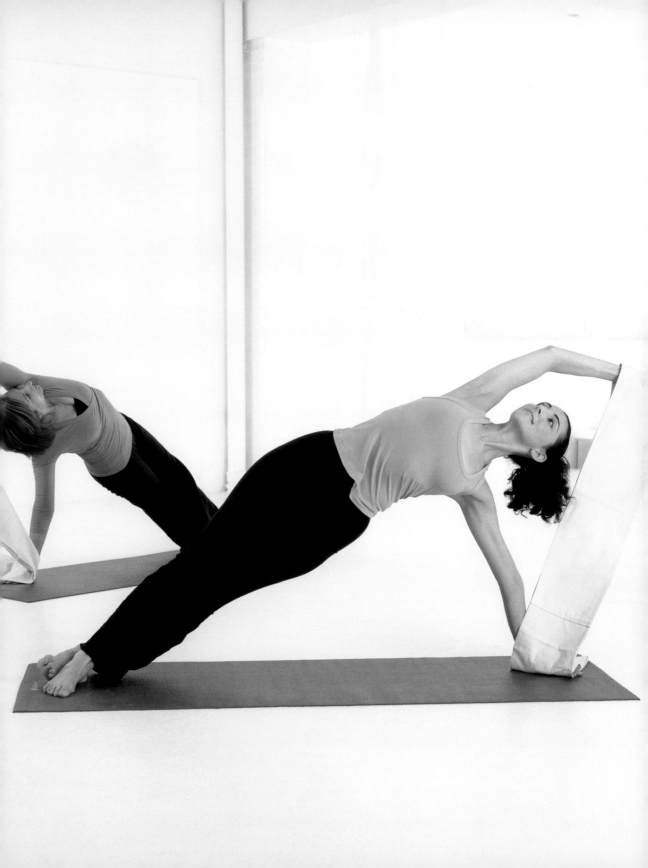

kneeling press with arm extensions

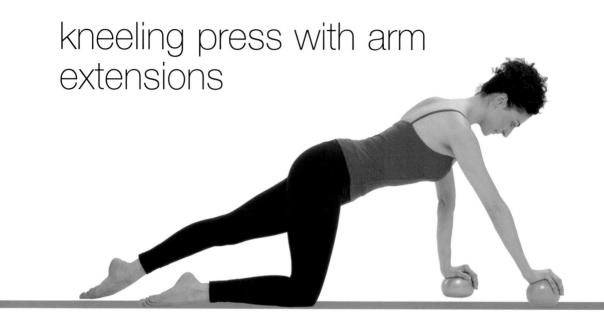

Benefits Coordination and balance play a major role in core fitness. Your strength system needs to be connected and centered for your kinetic energy to flow. This movement pattern trains your body to work more harmoniously.

Starting alignment Kneel on your hands and knees, holding your weights in your hands. Form a straight line from your shoulders to your hands and from your hips to your knees.

Movement sequence

1   Stretch one leg out straight behind your torso on the floor while stretching your opposite arm on the floor in front of you.

2   Lift your extended arm and leg up to shoulder and hip level. Keep your palm down.

3   Lower your arm and leg to the floor.

4   Lift and lower 5 times.

5   Bend your extended leg. Turn your palm to face upward and simultaneously bend your arm. Both your arm and leg bend only to 90 degrees, forming right angles.

6   Bend and extend 5 times.

7   Place your extended arm and leg on the floor. Keep your hips level and lower your torso to sit on your heel. Keep your opposite arm straight and the weight on the floor as you lower.

8   Lift your torso to the hands-and-knees position.

9   Perform this movement 5 times.

Repetitions Go through the sequence 2 times, alternating sides.

Breathing pattern Exhale as you lift your weights. Inhale as you lower.
Exhale as you bend your arm and leg.
Inhale as you extend.

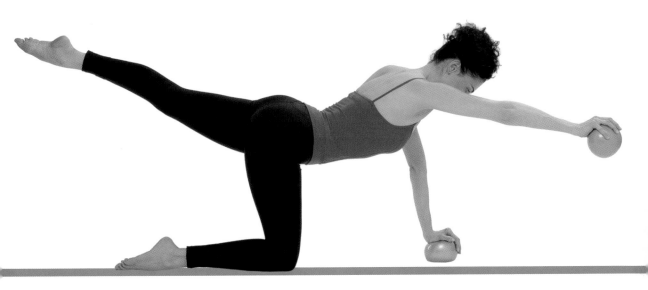

Exhale as you sit on your heel.

Inhale as you lift.

Goal Balanced hips and shoulders are your goal. Do not allow your core alignment to change at its source. Keep equal weight and height at all four points of your shoulders and hips. Make sure not to lean to one side.

Modifications Perform the entire pattern without using the weights.

Take the core challenge Pick up your pace and use sharp, precise movements as you curl your arm. Move quickly to change from the arm movement to sitting on your heel. Keep your core form as you move swiftly through the pattern.

kneeling washerwoman

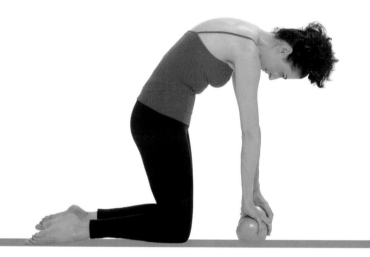

Benefits This exercise works your upper back, chest, and arms. As ever, the key to this exercise is forming a stable core.

Starting alignment Kneel on your mat, holding your hand weights. Round your torso forward and place the weights on the floor. Imagine that you are rounding over a large ball. Do not lean back or hunch your shoulders upward.

Movement sequence

1   Maintain your body design and pull your weights up from the floor, keeping your arms straight. Lift only a few inches from the floor.

2   Lower the weights to the floor then repeat this lift 5 times.

3   Lift a few inches from the floor. Bend your arms and pull your weights up to your chest, with elbows out to the side.

4   Lower your arms then repeat this lift 5 times.

5   Turn your palms to face inward. Bend your arms and lift your elbows to shoulder level.

6   Extend your arms behind your torso.

7   Bend your arms.

8   Repeat this movement 5 times.

9   Lower your arms and round your torso up.

Repetitions Go through the sequence once.

Breathing pattern Exhale as you pull your weights up from the floor.

Inhale to lower the weights to the floor.

Exhale as you bend your arms and pull your weights up to your chest.

Inhale to lower your arms.

Exhale as you extend your arms behind your torso.

Inhale when you bend your arms.

Take a full breath to round your torso up.

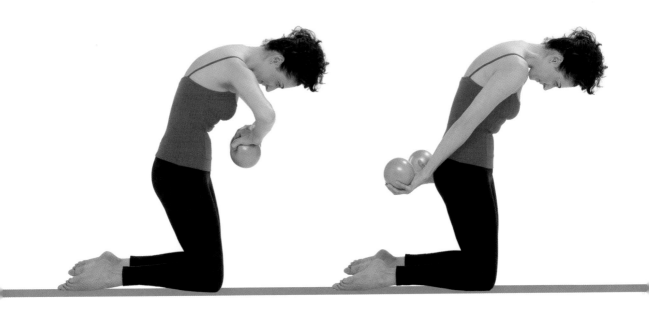

Goal Training your muscles with the principles of overload and specificity (see page 20) while maintaining core alignment will help you reach your goals faster and with less risk of strain. Work slowly and keep breathing deeply and consciously to avoid muscle stiffness. Keep your shoulders down and do not tense your neck muscles. Core alignment is key to performing this exercise properly. If you release your abdominal muscles, you will be putting tension into your lower back.

Modifications Perform this sequence without weights, if necessary.

Take the core challenge When you can complete 2 full sequences easily, it is time to add more weight.

kneeling mermaid with chest opening

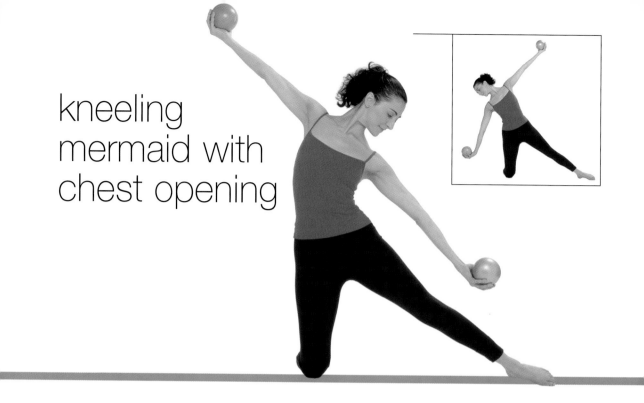

Benefits This exercise tones your obliques and helps create core stability for rotational movements. It will improve your spinal flexibility.

Starting alignment Kneel on your mat, holding your hand weights. Extend one leg out at the side of your body. Lift your arms up and bring them out at the side of your body to shoulder level.

Movement sequence: Kneeling Mermaid

1 Stretch your torso toward your outstretched leg, reaching your hand toward your foot.

2 Lift your torso up to the center position.

3 Keeping your arms lifted to shoulder level, stretch your torso away from your outstretched leg foot, reaching toward the floor at the opposite side of your body.

4 Lift into the center position and then repeat this pattern 5 times.

Movement sequence: Chest Opening

1 Place your hand on the floor next to your bent knee for support.

2 Lift your other arm to the ceiling.

3 Bring your top arm down to touch your supporting arm, rotating your torso toward the floor.

4 Lift your arm up to the ceiling, open your chest, and twist your torso to the back of the room.

5 Bring your top arm down and then repeat this pattern 5 times.

Repetitions Perform the series once on each side.

Breathing pattern: Kneeling Mermaid

Inhale to stretch your torso toward your leg.

Exhale as you lift your torso up.

Inhale as you stretch your torso away from your foot.

Exhale to lift into the center position.

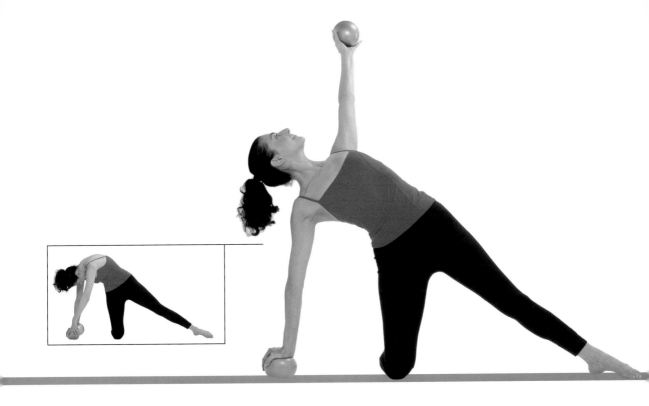

Breathing pattern: Chest Opening

Inhale and lift your arm to the ceiling.

Exhale as you rotate your torso toward the floor.

Inhale to open your chest and twist your torso.

Exhale and bring your top arm down.

Goal Make sure not to let your shoulders tip forward when you stretch side to side. They must remain directly over your hips. When doing the rotational part of this movement pattern, do not let your arm droop. Keep your arm next to your ear so your torso gets the maximum benefit of the work. Work from your core, twisting your torso before you lift your arm. Your arm should follow the movement, not lead it. If your arm leads the exercise, you will not be rotating your deep core muscles.

Modifications Perform the exercise without your weights to feel how your core muscles work.

heel sit

Benefits This is a wonderful exercise for toning your shoulder and arm muscles.

Starting alignment Kneel on your mat and sit on your heels. Hold your hand weights and place your arms down at the sides of your body. Keep your shoulders directly over your hips.

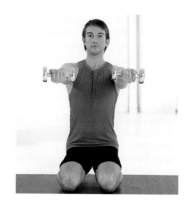

Movement sequence

1   Lift your arms up to chest level in front of your torso.
2   Bend your arms to your chest as you press your torso up to the kneeling position.
3   Sit on your heels, extending your arms out in front of your chest.
4   Repeat the movement 5 times.
5   Lift your torso up to kneeling, pulling your arms to your chest.
6   Extend your arms and pull them to your chest 10 times.
7   Sit on your heels, extending your arms out in front of your chest.
8   Lower your arms.

Repetitions Go through the movement pattern once.

Breathing pattern Inhale to lift your arms up to chest level.

Exhale as you bend your arms to your chest.

Inhale to sit on your heels.

Exhale as you lift your torso up to kneeling.

Inhale when you extend your arms.

Exhale to pull them to your chest.

Inhale as you sit on your heels.

Exhale to lower your arms.

Goal Keep your torso straight. Do not lean forward to press up or sit down. Make sure your arm movements are initiated from core strength and keep your shoulder alignment.

Modifications Stay seated on your heels and work your arms and chest muscles.

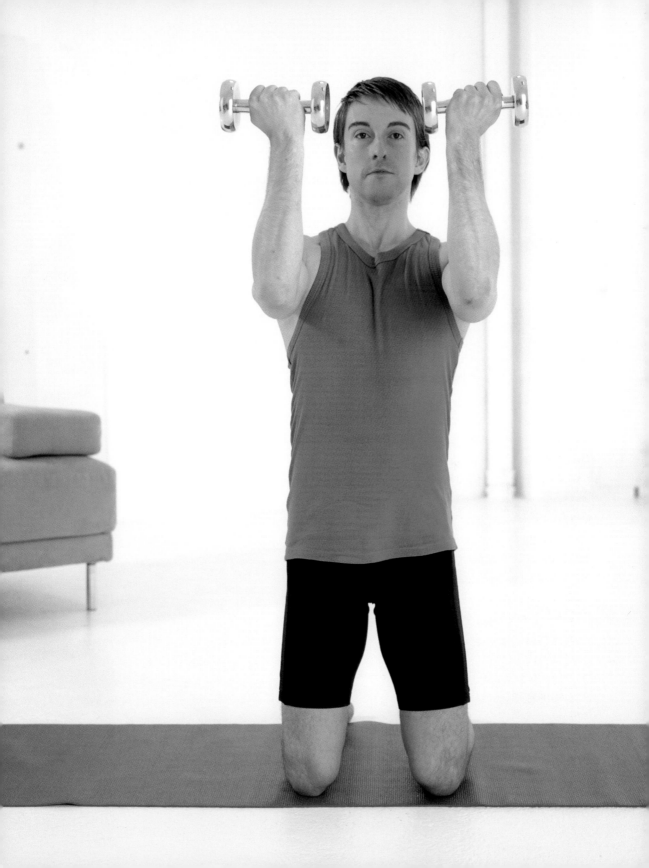

plank curls

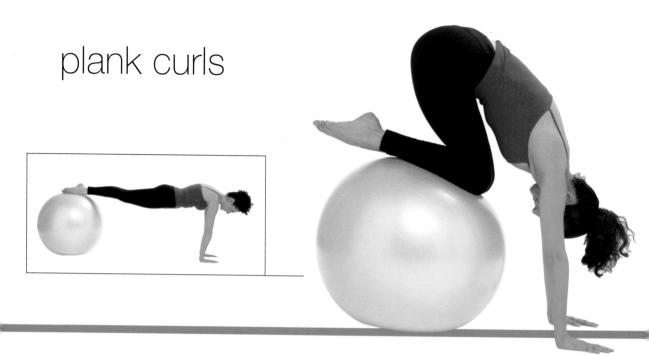

Benefits This exercise strengthens your abdominals, hips, and thighs. It is a great balancer for your inner core and internal organs. It's a challenging exercise, and not for the faint-hearted, but once you get the hang of it, you will feel the benefits.

Starting alignment Lie over your stability ball with your hands and feet on the floor.

Movement sequence

1 Lift your legs up to hip level. Walk your hands out until the ball is under your knees, bringing your body to a plank position.

2 Bending your knees and your hips, pull the ball under you until you are sitting on your heels.

3 Extend your legs out, returning to the plank position.

Repetitions Repeat the exercise 10 times.

Breathing pattern Inhale to walk your hands out.

Exhale as you sit on your heels.

Inhale as you extend your legs.

Goal Your goal is a perfect plank position at the start. Maintaining your core alignment is difficult in the fully extended position, but this is the goal. Check your cross-point alignment and initiate the curl from your lower abdominal muscles. Do not let your hips release or your back arch in the extended position. Keep your arms straight with your hands placed directly under your shoulders. Do not lean into your hands but keep your body weight held up in your core. Exhale deeply as you pull the ball under you to activate you abdominal muscles to begin the roll. Do not pull with your legs or push with your arms.

Take the core challenge Reverse the movement, stretching back until your arms are extended on the floor. Alternate rolling front and back.

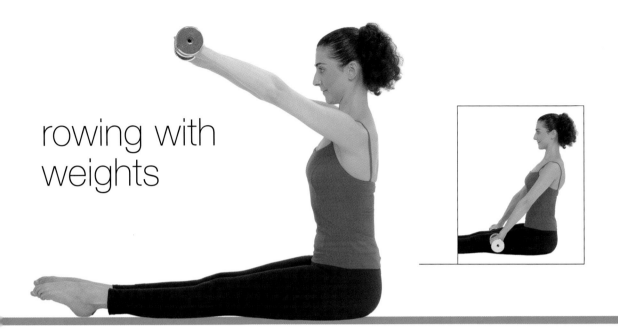

rowing with weights

Benefits The benefits to your upper back, chest, and arm muscles are complemented by the stabilization of your core muscles in this exercise.

Starting alignment Sit on your mat with your legs extended in front of you. Hold your hand weights with your palms facing down. Bend your elbows and bring them to your waist at the sides of your body. Sit tall with your spine straight.

Movement sequence

1 Extend your arms in front of your torso on a diagonal line to eye level.

2 Lower your arms to the floor at the sides of your body.

3 Lift your arms toward the ceiling, keeping them next to your ears.

4 Circle your arms out to the sides of your body to shoulder level with your palms down.

5 Bend your elbows and bring the weights in at your waist.

Repetitions Repeat the sequence 5 times.

Breathing pattern Inhale as you extend your arms on the diagonal line.

Exhale as you lower your arms to the floor.

Inhale as you lift your arms overhead.

Exhale as you circle your arms and bend them in.

Goal Keep your shoulders down and back lifted. Increase your range of motion by stabilizing your shoulders and working with smooth, fluid movements. Do not sink into your hips. Keep your head in line with your spine and your spine straight as if you were sitting up against a wall

Modifications Perform the movement without the weights, concentrating on a full range of motion with your arms while your torso remains still.

twist over the stability ball

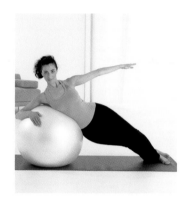

Benefits This versatile exercise works your obliques, back muscles, and abdominals all at once.

Starting alignment Stand with the ball to the right side of your body. Bend your knees and press your right hip and waist into the ball. Place your left foot in front of your right foot. Place your right hand on the ball and bring your left arm out at shoulder level.

Movement sequence

1 Stretch out, straightening your legs. Place your right hand on the floor as you stretch and lift your left arm toward the ceiling.

2 Bend your knees and lift your arm from the floor to release.

Repetitions Repeat 5 times.

Breathing pattern Inhale as you stretch over the ball. Exhale as you bend your knees.

Goal Your goal is to keep your hips and shoulders aligned as you stretch. Do not allow your hips or shoulders to twist forward or back.

Modifications Keep your bottom leg bent on the floor. Extend your top leg out. Stretch your torso over the ball and lift up.

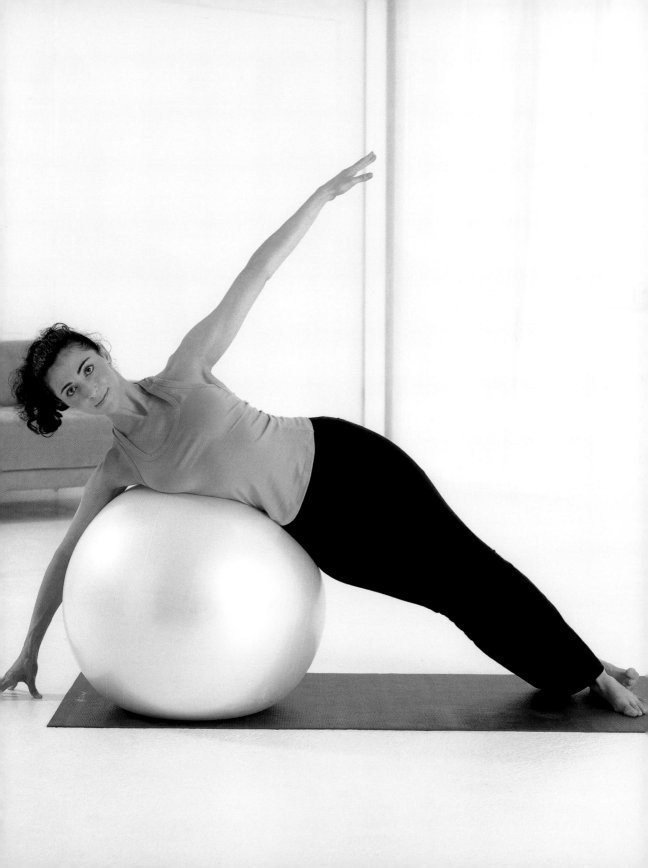

arm offering, salute, and shave your head

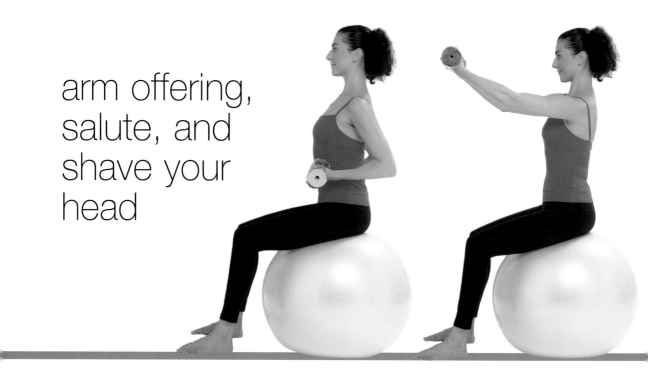

Benefits Well-toned arms and a strong upper body aid everyday activities. These three exercises form a very effective sequence that helps balance the muscle groups in your arms for functional strength. Sitting on your stability ball ensures that your core muscles are fully activated, but if you do not have a stability ball, you can perform the exercises without.

Starting alignment Hold your hand weights and sit on top of your stability ball. Place your feet on the floor, hip-distance apart. Bend your elbows and bring them to your waist at the sides of your body with your palms up. Sit tall with your spine straight and your core muscles activated. If you do not have a stability ball, perform these exercises sitting on the floor, with your legs extended straight in front of you.

Movement sequence: Arm Offering

1 Extend your arms in front of your torso on a diagonal line to eye level, keeping your palms facing up.

2 Bend your elbows in at your waist. Repeat the exercise 5 times.

Movement sequence: Salute

1 Extend your arms in front of your torso on a diagonal line to eye level, turning your palms down.

2 Bend your arms and bring your hands to your eyebrows like a salute. Repeat this movement 5 times.

Movement sequence: Shave Your Head

1 Hinge your torso forward, while keeping your back very straight. Bring your elbows next to your ears.

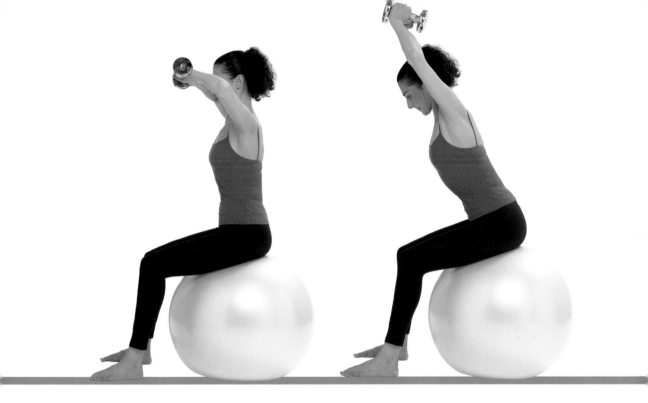

2   Bend your arms, bringing your hands behind your
    head. Repeat this movement pattern 5 times.

Repetitions Repeat the entire sequence 2 times.

Breathing pattern Inhale as you extend your
arms for all three exercises.

Exhale as you bend your arms.

Goal Your goal is a solid core with a good range of
arm movement. Keeping your hips and shoulders
balanced, hinge only as far as you can without
releasing your rib cage alignment.

Modifications Minimize the number of repetitions of
each movement, but do all three variations.

plow
Halasana

Benefits This whole-body stretch is found in many exercise regimes. Each variation has the same goal—total body strength and flexibility.

Starting alignment Lie on your mat. Bring your arms to your sides, palms down.

Movement sequence

1. Bend your knees toward your chest and extend your legs toward the ceiling over your hips.
2. Stretch your legs over your head, rolling your spine from the floor, one vertebra at a time.
3. Stretch back until your legs are parallel to the floor and your hips are over your shoulders. Support your back with your hands, if necessary.
4. Lower your feet to the floor.
5. Slowly roll your spine onto your mat, one vertebra at a time.

Repetitions Perform the Plow pose 3 times.

Breathing pattern Take a full breath as you roll back. Inhale and exhale as you place your feet on the floor. Stay in the pose for 3 full breaths. Roll down to your mat with 3 long, full breaths.

Goal Stretch fully from your core. Do not roll onto your neck but keep your weight in your shoulders and arms. Control the movement from your torso and activate your abdominals to support your back.

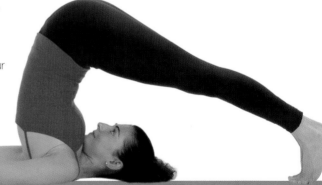

shoulderstand
Sarvangasana

Benefits This challenging pose benefits your heart and lungs and improves circulation. It should not be performed if you are pregnant.

Starting alignment Lie on your back with your legs extended and your hands at the sides of your body with your palms down.

Movement sequence

1 Bend your knees toward your chest and extend your legs over your head in Plow pose (see opposite).

2 Slowly lift your legs toward the ceiling, stretching from your shoulders to your hips to your toes. If necessary, support your back with your hands.

3 Stretch your legs overhead again and place your feet on the floor.

4 Roll your spine to your mat one vertebra at a time.

Repetitions Perform 3 repetitions of the Shoulderstand pose.

Breathing pattern Inhale as you bend your knees.

Exhale to extend your legs.

Take a complete breath to lift your legs into Plow.

Inhale and exhale to lift your legs toward the ceiling.

Hold the pose for 3 full breaths.

Inhale and exhale to place your feet on the floor.

Roll your spine to your mat with 3 more breaths.

Goal Stretch from your shoulders to your toes in one long, straight line. Keep your neck elongated on the floor and support your body weight in your shoulders.

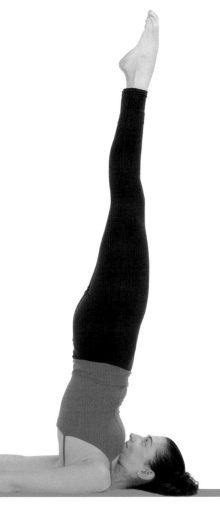

sun salutation

Benefits Sequencing is very important for the body to receive balanced muscle work. The Sun Salutation exemplifies the beauty of movement in action.

Starting alignment Stand with your feet together and your arms down at your sides. Align your body from the strong and rooted placement of your feet through your legs, core, and up to the top of your head. Breathe and center yourself before beginning your movement.

Movement sequence

1　Lift your arms over your head.
2　Round over into a standing forward bend.
3　Bend your knees and extend your left leg behind you into a lunge position.
4　Extend your left leg back to stretch your torso into a plank position.
5　Lower your torso into a push-up position.
6　Bring your feet hip-distance apart. Lengthen your spine in extension, arching upward from the floor.
7　Press your hips to the ceiling, pushing back with your straight arms and pushing your heels to the floor with legs straight. Concentrate on elongating your spine.
8　Step your left foot forward into a lunge position.
9　Step your right foot forward and straighten your legs. Stretch your torso toward your legs in a standing forward bend.
10 Stretch up to standing, lifting your arms overhead. You are now ready to begin the sequence again.

Repetitions Go through the entire sequence once or twice.

Breathing pattern Inhale to lift your arms over your head.
Exhale to round over. Take a full breath as you stretch.
Exhale to lunge. Inhale and lunge deeper.
Exhale into a plank position as you lower your torso.
Take 3 full breaths to arc up from the floor and lower down to your mat.
Exhale to lift and straighten your legs.
Take 3 breaths in this position.
Exhale as you lunge. Inhale as you increase your stretch.
Exhale as you step forward and straighten your legs.
Take a full breath to stretch in a forward bend.
Inhale to stretch up to standing.
Exhale and lower your arms.

Goal Move fluidly and with controlled precision, keeping your abdominals lifted and breathing deeply and consciously throughout the sequence.

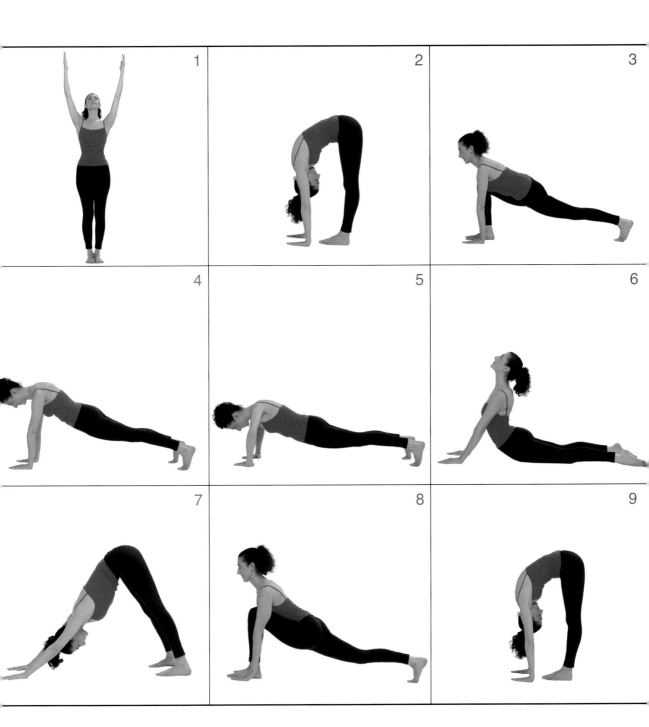

1

2

3

4

5

6

7

8

9

workout programs for life

10-MINUTE STRETCHING WORKOUT ▶

 Core Imprint, p38 ▶

 Reclining Leg Stretch, p46

 Lying Thigh over Thigh Twist, p47

 Lord of the Fishes, p45

 Kneeling Side Stretch, p94

 Stability Ball Pelvic Curls, p108

 Stability Ball Imprint, p116

 Stability Ball Swan, p117

 Twist with Arm Pulls, p122

 Neck and Shoulder Stretch, p80

 Side Stretch with Cross Reach, p83

 Standing Roll-down, p84

10-MINUTE DAILY MAINTENANCE WORKOUT ▶

 Diamond Contractions, p43 ▶

 The Hundred, p56

 Reclining Leg Stretch, p46

 Deltoid Fly, p100

 Ab Curls with Arm Extensions, p102

 Heel Sit, p138

 Kneeling Washer-woman, p134

 Side Kick Series, p63

 The Bridge, p125

 Tree Pose, p73

 Standing Side Bend, p78

 Standing Forward Bend, p74

20-MINUTE STRETCH AND TONE WORKOUT ▶

 Chest Expansion, p36 ▶

 Cobbler's Pose, p44

 Rolling Like a Ball, p58

 Single Leg Stretch, p60

 Double Leg Stretch, p61

 Head to Knee Pose, p68

 Seated Twist, p67

 The Saw, p86

 Open Leg Rocker, p87

 Roll-over, p88

 The Swan, p92

 Swimming, p93

 Straight Leg Lifts in Plank Position, p110

 Leg Extensions, p113

 Leg Twists, p109

 Seated Twist, p67

 Hip Circles, p123

 The Boomerang, p126

 Kneeling Mermaid, p136

 Kneeling Press with Arm Extensions, p132

 Forward Lunge with Biceps Curl, p50

 Side Bends with Straight Arm Lifts, p99

 Quadriceps Bend and Stretch, p52

 Hip, Thigh, and Leg Stretch, p54

 Tree Pose, p73

Standing Forward Bend, p74

Triangle Pose 1, p76

Mountain Pose, p72

20-MINUTE MAT WORKOUT ▶

 Core Imprint, p38 ▶

 Small Leg Circles, p40

 Large Leg Circles, p41

 Reclining Leg Stretch, p46

 Lying Thigh over Thigh Twist, p47

 The Hundred, p56

 Rolling Like a Ball, p58

 Single Leg Stretch, p60

 Double Leg Stretch, p61

 Side Kick Series, p63

 The Saw, p86

 Open Leg Rocker, p87

 Roll-over, p88

 The Swan, p92

 Swimming, p93

 The Teaser, p90

 Ab Curls with Arm Extensions, p102

 Oblique Curls with Arm Extensions, p104

 Seated Twist, p67

 Hip Circles, p123

 The Twist, p130

 Kneeling Press with Arm Extensions, p132

 Kneeling Washerwoman, p134

 Kneeling Mermaid, p136

 Heel Sit, p138

 Rowing with Weights, p141

 Arm Offering, Salute & Shave Your Head, p144

 Sun Salutation, p148

20-MINUTE FIT AND FLEX WORKOUT ▶

 Cobbler's Pose, p44 ▶

 Lord of the Fishes, p45

 Lying Thigh over Thigh Twist, p47

 Reclining Leg Stretch, p46

 Mountain Pose, p72

 Tree Pose, p73

 Standing Forward Bend, p74

 Standing Side Bend, p78

 Quadriceps Bend and Stretch, p52

 Hip, Thigh, and Leg Stretch, p54

 Seated Twist, p67

 Head to Knee Pose, p68

 Cobra Pose, p106

 Bow Pose, p107

 Stability Ball Pelvic Curls, p108

 Leg Twists, p109

 Straight Leg Lifts in Plank Position, p110

 Leg Extensions, p113

 Stability Ball Imprint, p116

 Stability Ball Swan, p117

 Spine Stretch and Twist, p118

 Push-ups and Leg Beats, p120

 The Boomerang, p126

 Plank Curls, p140

 Twist over the Stability Ball, p142

 Plow, p146

 Shoulder-stand, p147

 Sun Salutation, p148

60-MINUTE TOTAL BODY WORKOUT ▶

 Chest Expansion, p36 ▶

 Core Imprint, p38

 Small Leg Circles, p40

 Large Leg Circles, p41

 Diamond Contractions, p43

 Cobbler's Pose, p44

 Reclining Leg Stretch, p46

 Lying Thigh over Thigh Twist, p47

 Forward Lunge with Biceps Curl, p50

 Quadriceps Bend and Stretch, p52

 Hip, Thigh, and Leg Stretch, p54

 The Hundred, p56

 Rolling Like a Ball, p58

 Single Leg Stretch, p60

 Double Leg Stretch, p61

 Reclined Twist, p66

 Seated Twist, p67

 Mountain Pose, p72

 Tree Pose, p73

 Standing Forward Bend, p74

 Triangle Pose 1, p76

 Triangle Pose 2, p77

 Standing Side Bend, p78

 Neck and Shoulder Stretch, p80

Side Stretch with Cross Reach, p83

Standing Roll-down, p84

The Saw, p86

Open Leg Rocker, p87

Roll-over, p88

 The Swan, p92

 Swimming, p93

 Kneeling Side Stretch, p94

 Side Bends with Biceps Curls, p97

 Side Bends with Straight Arm Lifts, p99

 Deltoid Fly, p100

 Ab Curls with Arm Extensions, p102

 Oblique Curls with Arm Extensions, p104

 Cobra Pose, p106

 Bow Pose, p107

 Stability Ball Pelvic Curls, p108

 Straight Leg Lifts in Plank Position, p110

 Leg Extensions, p113

 Leg Twists, p109

 Stability Ball Swan, p117

 Push-ups and Leg Beats, p120

 Twist with Arm Pulls, p122

 Hip Circles, p123

 The Boomerang, p126

 Kneeling Side Kicks, p128

 The Bridge, p125

 The Twist, p130

 Plank Curls, p140

 Twist over the Stability Ball, p142

 Rowing with Weights, p141

 Arm Offering, Salute & Shave Your Head, p144

 Sun Salutation, p148

index

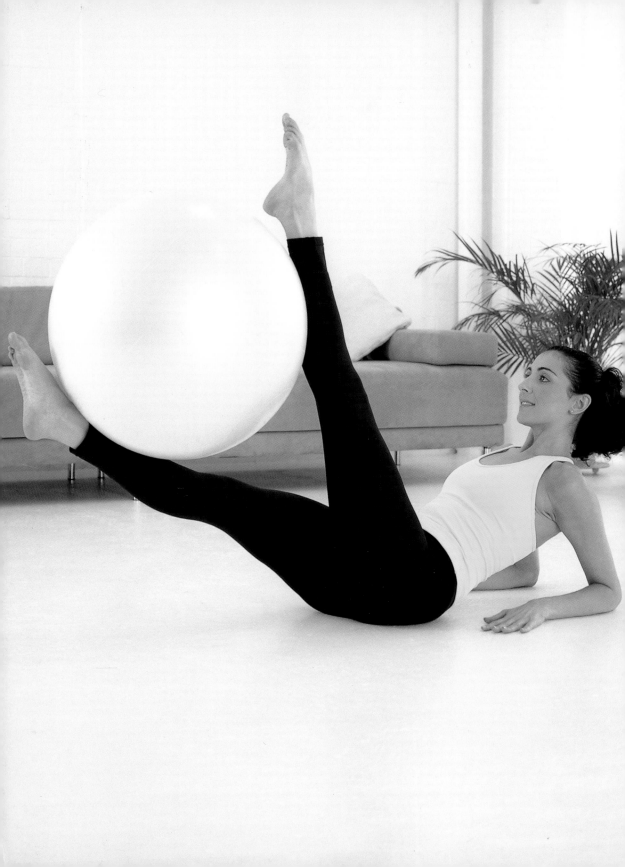